pink
power intensity naturally kindled
yoga

pink yoga

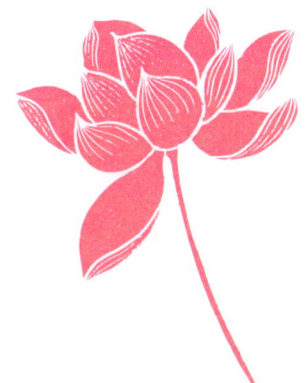

CP Sharma
Commander (Retd.)

RUPA

Copyright © CP Sharma (Commander Retd.) 2011

Published 2011 by
Rupa Publications India Pvt. Ltd.
7/16 Ansari Road, Daryaganj
New Delhi 110 002

Sales Centres:
Allahabad Bengaluru Chennai
Hyderabad Jaipur Kathmandu
Kolkata Mumbai

All rights reserved
No part of this publication may be
reproduced, stored in a retrieval system,
or
transmitted in any form or by any means,
electronic, mechanical, photocopying,
recording or otherwise without the prior
permission of the Publishers.

The author asserts the moral right to be
identified as the author of this work.

Book design by Sonali Lal
(Sonalilal@gmail.com)

Printed in India by
Nutech Photolithographers
B-240, Okhla Industrial Area, Phase-I,
New Delhi 110 020, India

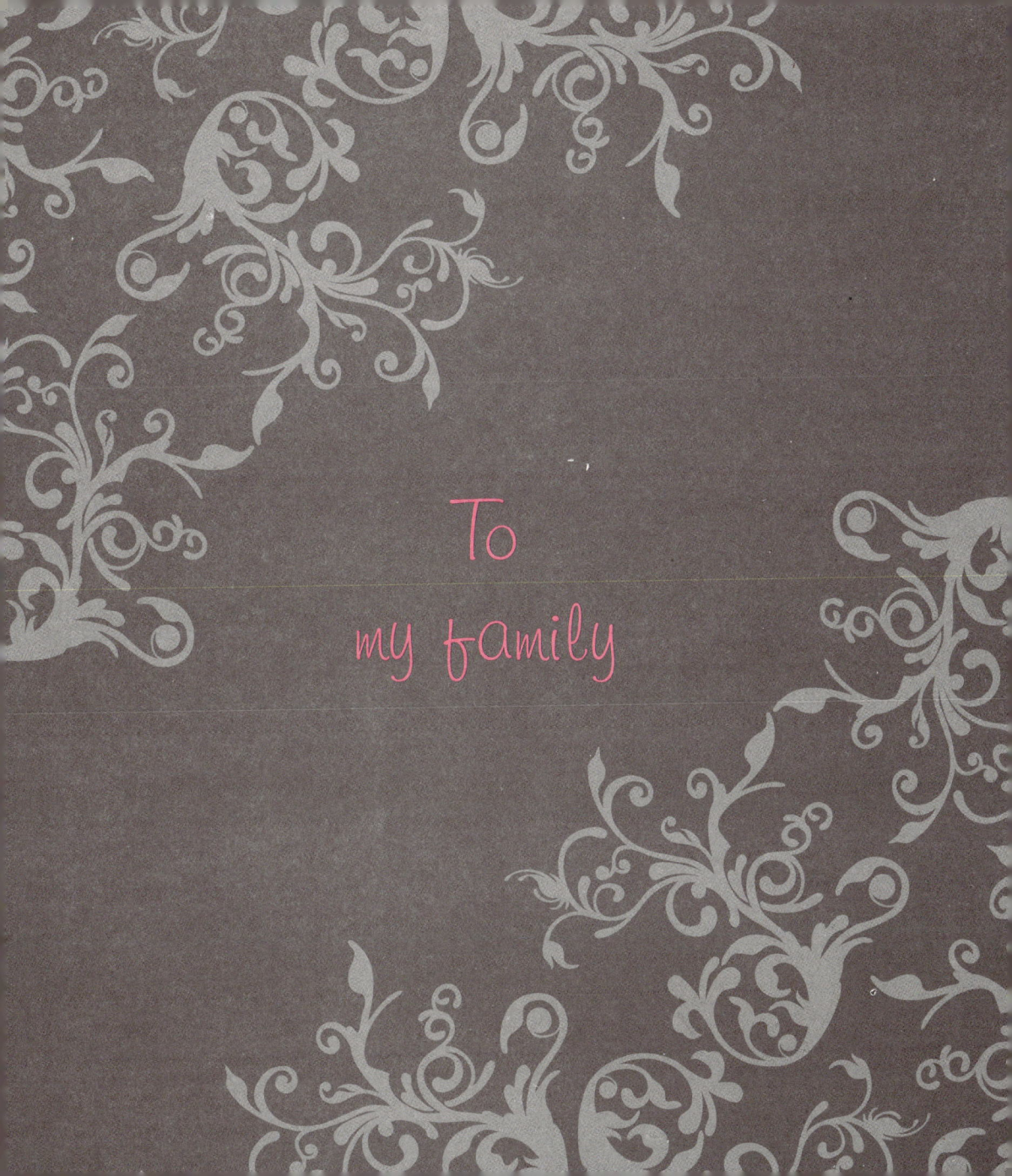

Contents

Foreword	ix
1. **Introduction**	1
2. **Our Body: Matter, Energy, Emotions**	3
3. **Modern Living and its side effects**	9
4. **To Good Health – Sex ... Vigour ... Vitality**	11
• Preservation & Restraint	11
• Yogic Discipline	13
• Asanas (Postures)	18
- Shavasana	18
- Padmasana	19
- Sukhasana	20
- Tadasana	21
- Surya Namaskar	22
- Vajrasan	26
- Gomukhasana	27
- Supta Vajrasana	28
- Shashankasana	29
- Vakrasana	30
- Bhujangasana	31

- - Kandharasan — 32
  - - Shalabhasana — 33
  - - Viparitakarani — 34
  - - Matsyasana — 35
- Pranayama (Breath Control) — 36
  - - Anulom Vilom / Nadi Shodhan — 38
  - - Ujjayi — 40
  - - Kapalbhati — 41
  - - Naad Yog — 42
  - - Yog Nidra : Yogic Sleep — 43
- Bandhs (Air Locks) — 45
  - - Jalandhar Bandh — 45
  - - Uddiyan Bandh — 46
  - - Mool Bandh — 47
  - - Maha Bandh — 47
- Meditation — 48
  - - Vibration Meditation — 50
  - - Movement Meditation — 51
- Kamasutric Art of Love — 53
- Dietary Advice — 65
- Acupressure — 69

5. **Therapeutic Applications and Common Problems** — 81

6. **Ideal Packages** — 87

7. **Acknowledgements** — 89

8. **Index** — 91

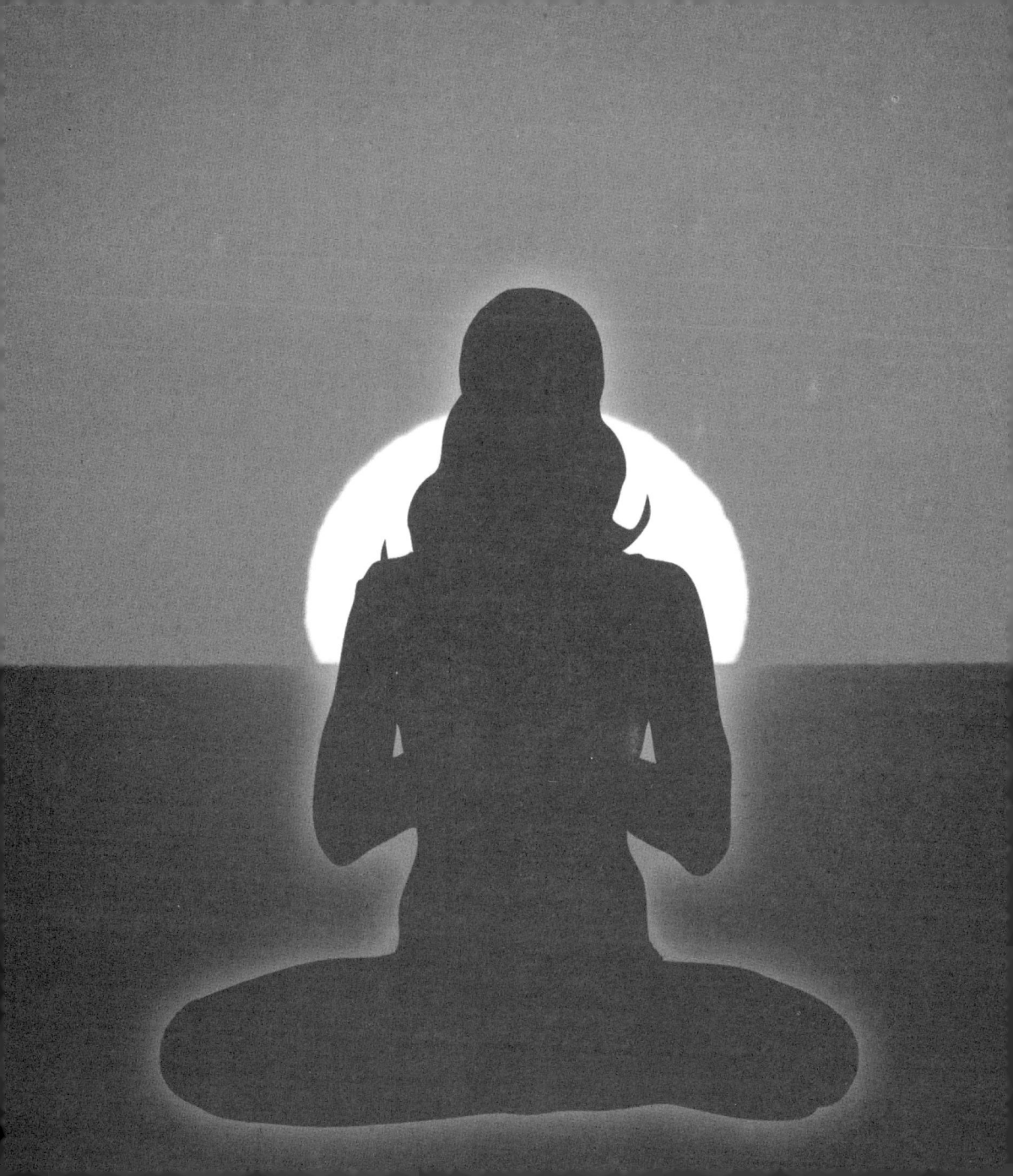

Foreword

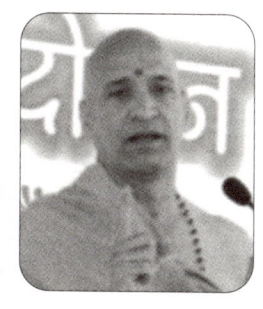

All the worldly activities of human beings find their reason around 'kama', which means *shakti* (power), the motivating force behind big achievements. Controlled *kama* is the pathway to miracles in human life while the excess of *kama* can irreversibly lead to destruction. Mythological beings like Hanuman and Bheeshma, and some great personalities like Swami Dayanand Saraswati and Swami Vivekananda are examples personifying controlled *kama*.

Kamashakti has a very important role to play in all the four *ashrams* of human life, *Brahmacharya*, *Grehastha*, *Vanaprastha* and *Sanyasa*. It is a general perception that when an individual indulges in *kama*, popularly known as sex, he surrenders to his lower instincts and loses the opportunities of attaining spiritual salvation. Even in the material world such people remain a failure because of unregulated sex and misapprehensions about it. This invariably leads to an escalation in malpractices and crime in society. In yoga *sadhana*, *kama* is considered the prime enemy among the six prominent enemies or obstacles in the way of spirituality: 1. *Kama* (sex) 2. *Krodh* (anger) 3. *Mad* (ego) 4. *Lobh* (greed) 5. *Moha* (ignorance) 6. *Matsar* (jealousy) on the path of *adhyatma sadhana*. These enemies hinder the progress of a yoga seeker. Thereby, it is advised that any avid yoga seeker on the path of spiritual bliss should protect oneself from these obstacles. Perhaps this has been the reason why brahmacharis lead such a difficult and restricted lifestyle.

I have been of the opinion that escape from reality is not the way to succeed. Living in denial can never be the solution to the problems of the world. For long, such restrictions could add nothing to the personalities of our youngsters. On the contrary, most of them are easily misled and often

pinkyoga

find themselves indulging in malpractices pertaining to sex. As *kama* has been considered the core enemy in the path of *Adhyatma Sadhna*, it becomes our duty to understand the enemy before devising a combat strategy. An aspirant should know the strength and weaknesses of the enemy to overpower it. Controlled *kama* may lead us to holistic development of our personality, improved strength and help greatly in attaining the higher stages of *sadhana*. Proper knowledge of *kama* can steer us clear of the prevalent confusions surrounding the same. Our youth is losing confidence, strength and stamina only because of improper knowledge and fears created by people who lack awareness of *kama*.

It is imperative to share proper knowledge with youngsters to prevent them from being misled and to make them understand the right use of *kamashakti* in everyday life. It is certainly the integral part of yoga and spiritual *sadhana*.

I am happy to learn that a former naval officer, Commander CP Sharma, after his deep study on the subject has successfully been able to write a book to impart proper yogic suggestions backed by scientific knowledge on the subject. Readers shouldn't simplistically treat this work as a sex book but as an ideal scientific and spiritual approach that removes confusions regarding *kamashakti* and helps one to stay youthful.

May the book guide people in the right direction and put an end to all misconceptions about *kama* and may it bring positive transformations in people of all ages.

Padmashri Bharat Bhushan
President
Mokshayatan International Yogashram, Saharanpur
www.bharatyog.com

'Sex and Health are two sides of the same coin.'

- Dr AK Jain
Renowned Sexologist

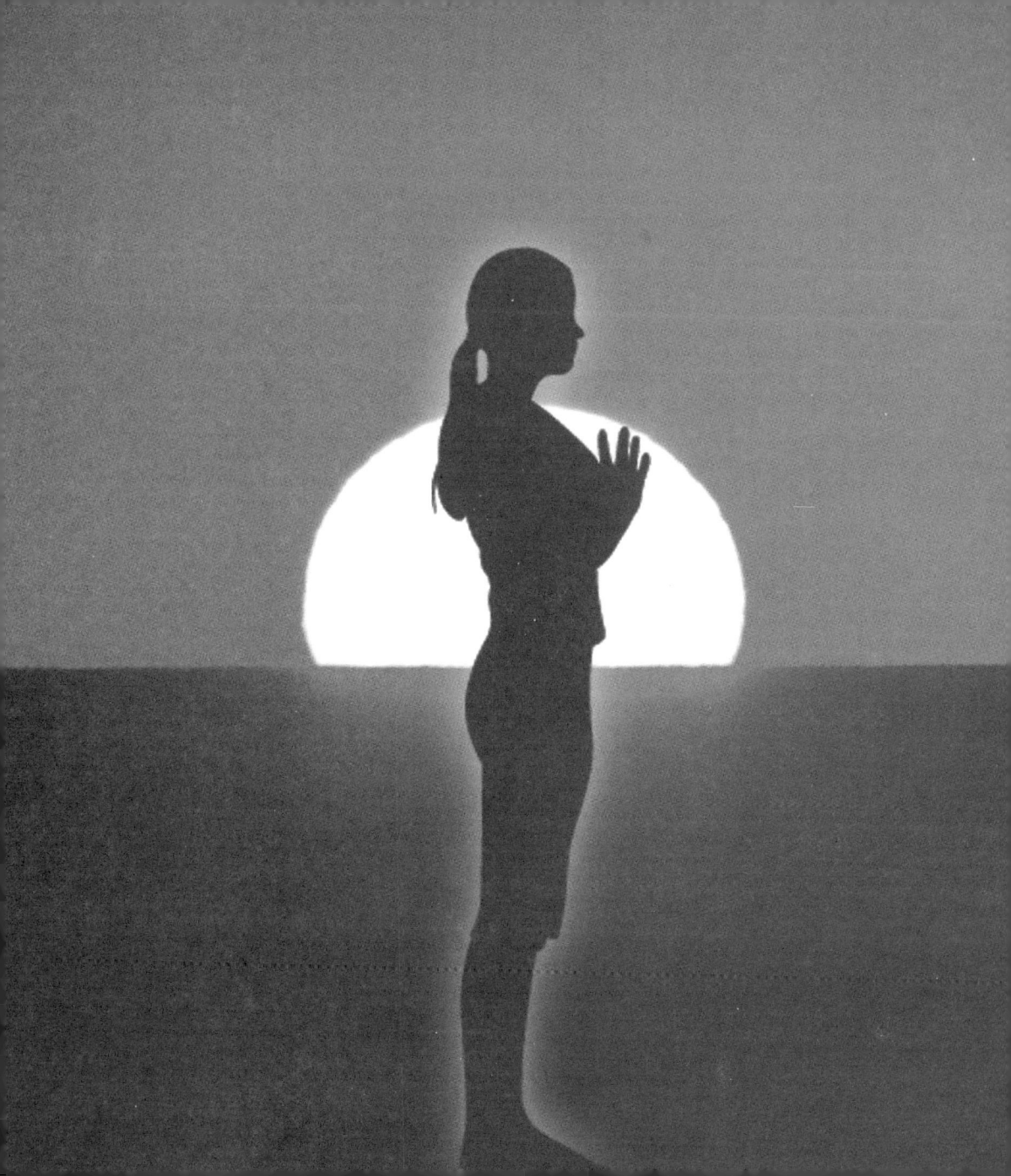

Introduction

Dear Reader,

For a moment please detach the social stigma of obscenity from the word 'sex' and let us consider what it in reality is and how the same should be perceived and studied.

Please ponder over the following facts:

- One of the aims of sexual union is procreation – the basic essence of life.

- A human being is considered relatively young as long as the sex hormonal secretions (SHS) continue to function normally.

- Women enjoy better health till menopause. Menopause is the time in a woman's life when the menstrual cycle ends, i.e. the stoppage of secretion of the hormone estrogen.

- In men as well prostrate problems do not make their presence felt as long as the secretion of the hormone, testosterone are normal.

- It is believed that regular sex keeps away obesity.

- Sex and health are two sides of the same coin. Only a healthy person is able to enjoy good sex. And sex gives both pleasure and health.

- Sex is a part of nature. Apart from giving physical pleasure it also helps in keeping away heart problems as it increases the heart rate and blood circulation, thereby providing better oxygen assimilation in the body.

- A human body expends approx. 114 Kcals during copulation. Besides, it also acts as a stress-reliever and anti-depressant. On the other hand if we were to burn these many calories through exercise, one would have to walk a minimum of 2.25 kms!

- The so-called erotic – actually erogenous – sculptures in some of the Hindu temples and even *Kamasutra* of Sage Vatsayayan should not be brushed aside as polluted philosophies. These are valuable knowledge banks and a pathway to healthy sexual life.

This book's aim is to clear the misconception and advise 'Yogic Discipline' and support therapies for individuals to keep them in good – almost perfect – health till possible; and maybe the entire life span.

2
Our Body – Matter, Energy, Emotions

The human body connects with the cosmos, the universe, through the electromagnetic fields. The energies that envelope, permeate or bombard humans are basically of three types:

- I. **Cosmic radiations:** Sun, Moon, and other planets
- II. **Telluric radiations:** Earth
- III. **Artificial radiations:** Man-made devices like TV, radio, radars, satellites, etc.

The ancient yogis in India even before Ayurveda emerged were aware of the internal energy sources generated and regulated by *chakras*, **'spinning wheels of energy'**, located at seven points along the spine of the body. The first is the crown *chakra* at the top of the head, and the last, the seventh is the root *chakra* at the base of the spine. There are also many minor *chakras* positioned around the body.

Correlating with the Western discoveries these correspond to the endocrine (ductless) glands, which are also regulators and protectors of the body mechanism. The internal secretions - called hormones - produced by the glands upon getting mixed with blood build-up, and help maintain the body in healthy condition.

The major *chakras* are associated with endocrine glands responsible for our identification with emotions, functions, colours and even musical notes. [*refer fig 1 and table on page 5*]

pinkyoga

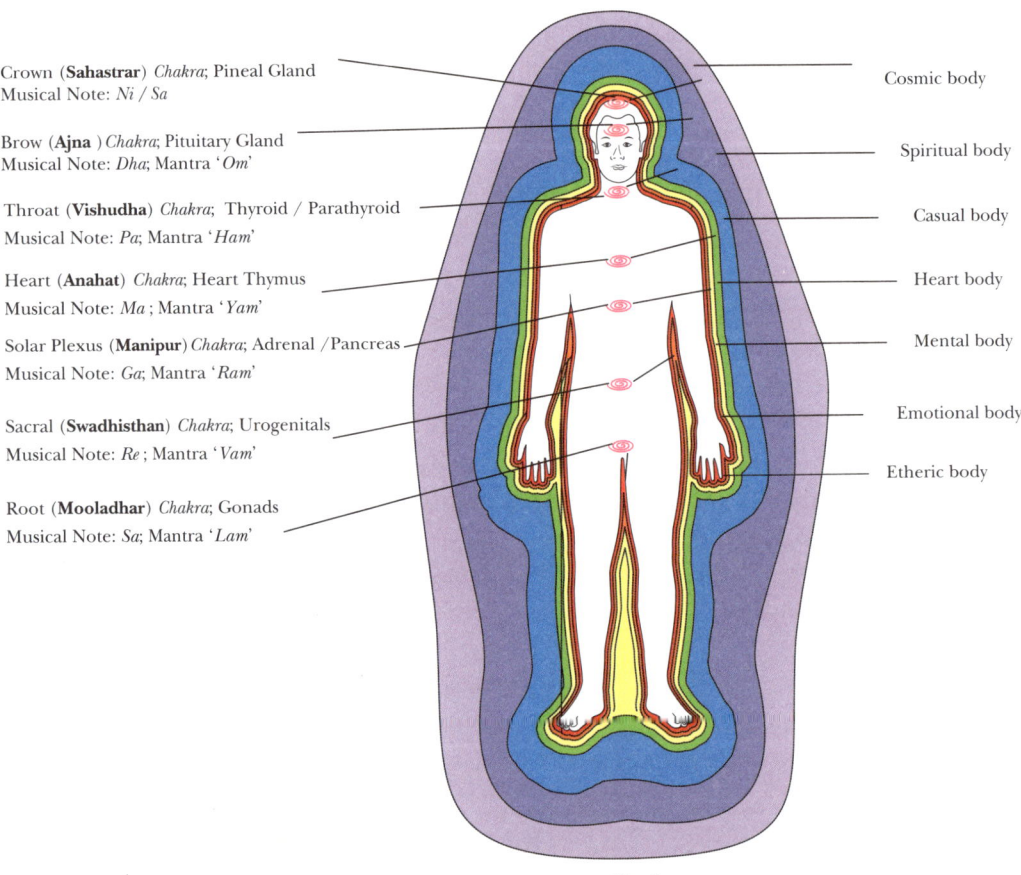

Crown (**Sahastrar**) *Chakra*; Pineal Gland
Musical Note: *Ni / Sa*

Brow (**Ajna**) *Chakra*; Pituitary Gland
Musical Note: *Dha*; Mantra '*Om*'

Throat (**Vishudha**) *Chakra*; Thyroid / Parathyroid
Musical Note: *Pa*; Mantra '*Ham*'

Heart (**Anahat**) *Chakra*; Heart Thymus
Musical Note: *Ma*; Mantra '*Yam*'

Solar Plexus (**Manipur**) *Chakra*; Adrenal /Pancreas
Musical Note: *Ga*; Mantra '*Ram*'

Sacral (**Swadhisthan**) *Chakra*; Urogenitals
Musical Note: *Re*; Mantra '*Vam*'

Root (**Mooladhar**) *Chakra*; Gonads
Musical Note: *Sa*; Mantra '*Lam*'

Cosmic body

Spiritual body

Casual body

Heart body

Mental body

Emotional body

Etheric body

Fig. 1

It is rightly said that our emotional state is often a barometer of our health. The following table helps in understanding the body sheath, its corresponding *chakra*, glands and organs along with the linked emotions.

Our Body – Matter, Energy, Emotions

S.No	Body Sheath	Corresponding *Chakra*	Corresponding Endocrine Gland/Organs	Linked Emotions and Functions
1.	Cosmic	*Sahastar* (Crown)	Pineal	**Spirituality; inspirations** • Manager of all glands; regulates water balance; controls sexual desires; stimulates nerves, growth.
2.	Spiritual	*Ajna* (Brow)	Pituitary	**Will; intuition** • Considered the king of all glands; growth of body, brain power and memory.
3.	Casual	*Vishudha* (Throat)	Thyroid/Parathyroid	**Communication; self expression** • Temperature regulation; energy production.
4.	Heart	*Anahat* (Heart)	Thymus	**Unconditional love** • Godmother till children reach 12-15 yrs of age.
5.	Mental	*Manipur* (Solar Plexus)	Adrenal / Pancreas	**Self-esteem** • Controls water balance; controls stress; helps in remaining active and character building.
6.	Emotional	*Swadhisthan* (Sacral)	Urogenitals	**Sexuality; creativity; action.** • Excretion and control of organs located below the diaphragm.
7.	Etheric	*Mooladhar* (Root)	Gonads (Ovaries / Testes)	**Material survival; elimination.** • Production of sex hormones; control of water and phosphorous content in the body.

Human actions/reactions, body language, character, diseases are all the outcome of interactivity of the body matter, energies around and above all, emotions. For example, any disease first affects the aura – the electromagnetic field around the body – and then descends on the body.

Emotions affect our health in a big way. Let us see how the tree of emotions ascends from *mooladhar* (root) to *sahastrar* (crown) *chakra* that is from 'Material Survival' to the bliss of 'Spirituality' *(refer Fig. 2)*.

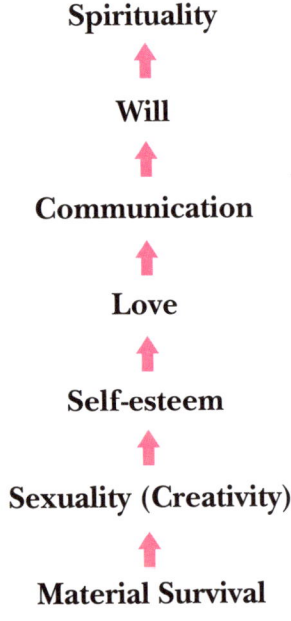

Fig. 2- The Tree of Emotions

According to Yoga, the latent energy called *kundalini* (serpentine) is stored at the root *chakra* and as it moves upwards, through certain yogic practices, the power of these glands is increased manifold; which in turn infuses relevant qualities in the human character and personality.

We can also say that emotional upheavals affect the 'energy' levels in the body which in turn affect the metabolism. The 'emotions' and 'hormonal secretions' directly affect each other. Hence, if stimulation / balancing of *chakras* can be managed, the same would automatically give impetus to our emotional strengths.

The *Mooladhar chakra* is the base plexus (with gonads location) and is responsible for sex hormonal secretions (SHS). Keeping the gonads/*chakra* well stimulated and maintaining proper levels of SHS in the body leads to healthier lifestyle, delayed andropause/menopause, and prolonged youth.

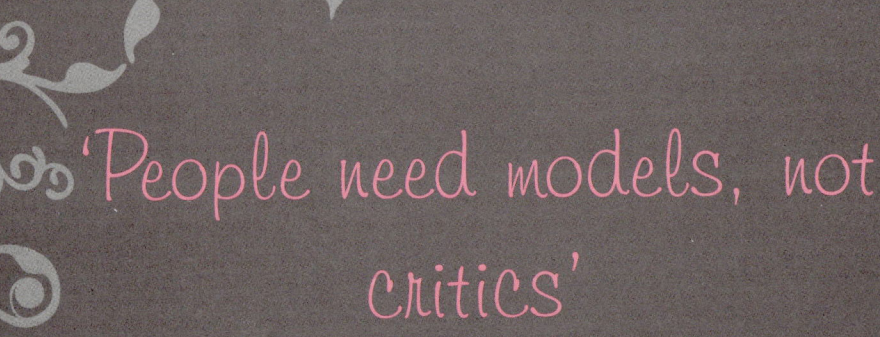

'People need models, not critics'

– John Wooden

3

Modern Living and its Side Effects

The hectic lifestyle of the current generation is, in short, the sum total of the following factors:

- Fast-paced
- Little 'tolerance' society
- Highly competitive work culture
- Nuclear families

People in the present society have moved from being 'nomadics' to 'settlers' with the emphasis being more on 'consumption' rather than 'conservation'! The advertisements aired/displayed today also seem to propagate the same philosophy. The mode of transport, communication, etc., have all become (super) fast; leaving little patience and at times even no patience at all in individuals. Cases of road rage, criminal tendencies are all on the rise and more visible today. It is difficult to sustain harmony and maintain equilibrium in such a scenario.

Life wasn't the same even a decade ago. With hectic lifestyles and 'no-time-for-anything' attitude, family relations have literally gone for a toss. Herein, the major setback has been for physical intimacy shared between couples. Because of long working hours and stress, couples often tend to regard sex also as part of their duty rather than enjoying it. This psychological lust, thus generated could lead to serious depression and perverted or unnatural sex; some even gaining acceptability in modern society.

A healthy and relaxed mind is important for mutually satisfying physical intimacy. The competitive environment is unlikely to change overnight; thereby it is advised to balance the emotional tree of our life, through strict yogic regimen. Sex should never be treated out of context as it plays an important role in bringing balance to an individual. It is believed that these acts induce partial release – being sensitive to SHS – of *kundalini* to travel upward through the spinal cord and act as 'emotion-booster-cum-tranquiliser'. If *mooladhar* and *swadhisthan chakras* are properly balanced, the upper emotions/ *chakras* automatically fall in line naturally.

Any science or methods that can harmonise the mind, body and soul can have perfect results on our body, its character, longevity and enjoyability. The following table shows how yogic approach is more 'complete' and appropriate to harmonise the mind, body and soul than normal exercising or gymming.

Physical Exercises	Yoga
• Dissipation and recharge of energy.	• Harnessing and rechannelling of energy.
• Muscles get stiff and require more oxygen/blood; reduced sustainability in age increases.	• Muscles get supple, firm and full of strength, sustainable even in old age.
• Heavy diets.	• Austere diets.
• The spinal system stiffens; the main cord of the body's connectivity and actuating mechanism.	• The spinal system remains flexible and keeps communication and other channels well connected & healthy.
• Does not stimulate brain and internal organs in a regimented manner – a sort of neglect is imbued.	• Stimulates the brain through a combination of Asanas/Pranayams and systematic channelling of energy.
• Requires lot of space/gadgets.	• Requires just a mat/rug of 4' X 6' size or more.

'Must you be on a vigorous exercise regime, always follow it up with a 35 minutes yoga session to achieve proportionate balance in the body.'

4

To Good Health – Sex…Vigour…Vitality

PRESERVATION… RESTRAINT… REPRODUCTIVE BIOLOGY

A clay pot if not baked properly can develop deformities if put to use. Similar is the case of humans, more so during adolescence.

Adolescence is the time period between the beginning of puberty and adulthood. It sets in around the age of 12 when (semen) sperms start multiplying and maturing in boys and a monthly cycle starts in girls. The 'preservation and maturing' process demands that the precious semen (वीर्य) in males and ova (रज) in females are not wasted till the age of atleast 21 and 18, respectively.

The tedious process of semen formation takes about 50 days and seven steps. Out of forty kgs of digested food one kg of blood is formed and only a few drops of semen are formed in the next 49 days as described in the following seven steps:

Liquid > Blood > Fat > Muscles > Bones > Bone Marrow > Semen

It is very important to maintain proper levels of semen in the body. If for some reason the level of semen goes down, due to excessive or early sex, it induces reverse process of damaging the bone marrow blood, which in turn slows down the generation of red blood cells (RBCs) and enough antibodies. The syndrome gets weakened and the overworked endocrine glands stop producing vital hormones; thereby the body becoming prone to **AIDS** (Acquired Immuno Deficiency Syndrome).

During the circulation of blood in the head, a fluid called **'cerebro spinal fluid'** is extracted from it. A very vital fluid called nectar by our yogis, it travels down through the spinal cord up to the prostate gland, generating electricity. This electrical energy gets stored as latent energy (the *kundalini* – serpentine energy) in prostate (in males) / in skene's gland (in females).

Further, as per reproductive biology, the egg of a female is -ve electricity and when spermatozoa (+ve) energy enters into it; a battery cell is created as shown:

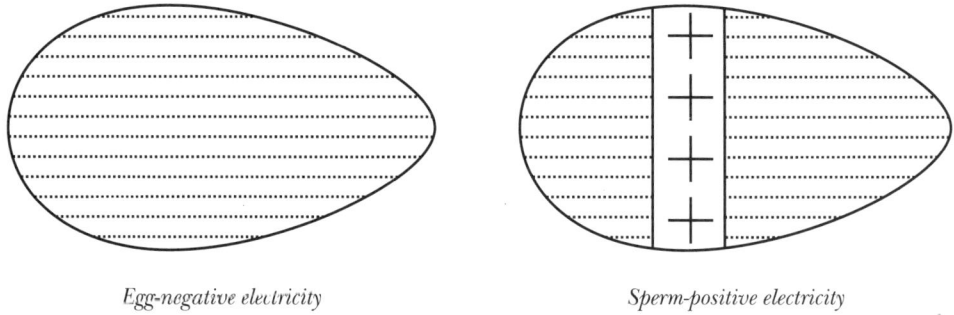

Egg-negative electricity *Sperm-positive electricity*

This (fertilised egg) battery cell eventually develops into a full grown human being expanding 60 billion times – probably the greatest wonder of cosmos.

YOGIC DISCIPLINE

The word 'Yoga' comes from the Sanskrit word *'yog'* meaning 'to join'. More aptly, it could be designated as 'fusion' and 'harmony' of the lower human nature with the higher in such a manner as to allow the higher to direct the lower or a combination of +ve and -ve energies or the union of *Shiva* and *Yoni* (male/female congress) or the union of *atma* (soul) and *parmatma* (Almighty).

Yoga doesn't propagate celibacy. It is a method to achieve 'bliss' and enjoy blissful living through all the various *ashrams* (phases) of life; be it 'restraint', 'indulgence' or 'seclusion' through these periods.

Yoga if practised earnestly can act as a dynamic balancer to human psychology. It can prevent diversion (perversion tendencies) because it balances the 'emotional tree'.

The most prevalent, practised and applicable yoga in our contemporary society is the:

Ashtang Yoga *(of eight steps)*

Yama — Moral discipline, i.e. truthfulness, non-killing, non-stealing.

Niyama — Cleanliness, contentment, austerity.

Asanas — Postures to reach higher state of physical and mental health.

Pranayam — Control of *prana* (breath).

pinkyoga

Pratyahar Restraint of senses from the objects.

Dharna Fixing the mind on a spot.

Dhyana Meditation.

Samadhi Superconsciousness.

The following guidelines should be kept in mind by practitioners before starting any yoga session:

- The best time to practice Yoga is on an empty stomach, ideally early morning before breakfast. At any other time, it should be done on a fairly empty stomach, i.e. two hours after a light meal or four hours after a heavy meal.

- Practice regularly for at least half-an-hour daily, preferably at the same time.

- Loose and comfortable clothing should be worn (proper underwear/*langoti* is a must).

- Practice with bare feet and on a blanket or a carpet to protect the body against earth's magnetism and to avoid any pricks from uneven grounds. **The ground should always be horizontal.**

- Practice in a warm, quiet, clean, dimly lit and airy place.

- Remove glasses and contact lenses before practice.

- Empty the bladder before practice.

- Avoid practising *asanas* during pregnancy (at least after 3 months of pregnancy) and during serious illness or high fever.

- In all *asanas* in which right or left side of the body is stretched more than the other, the balancing act on the other side must be done in a similar way.

- The *upasanas* (counter pose) should be done in recommended sets, e.g. locust posture after *bhujang*, *shashank* after *ushtra* or *supta vajrasana*, etc.

- *Asanas* must be done slowly, smoothly with full understanding and concentration on the recommended *chakra* / body part.

- Incorporate breathing while going into or coming out of the *asana*, as well as while holding of the *asana*. Breathe out during all forward bending movements in which the chest or the abdomen is being compressed, and breathe in during all backward bending movements in which the chest or abdomen is being expanded. The breath and the movement of going into and coming out of the *asanas* should be synchronised. Breathe normally while maintaining the pose, with full awareness / concentration on the technique of breathing.

- Coming out of the pose must be done by retracing the steps of going into the *asanas*.

- Do not force yourself into any final pose. Know your own limitations.

- If practising in a group, do not try to compete with others. Take your own time to complete the *asana*.

pinkyoga

- If you have any medical problem, consult your specialist doctor as well as inform your yoga teacher about the same.

- *Asanas* and *Pranayama* may be done after due modification by taking guidance from the yoga teacher in serious cardiovascular, respiratory, orthopaedic and other systemic disorders.

- A warm bath before and 15 minutes after the session will help people who suffer from arthritis.

- Beneficial effects will be observed after three months of regular and sincere practice and even more so after six months.

- The sequence during yogic session should be:
    - *shavasana*
    - *tadasana* (lying position).
    - standing postures
    - sitting postures
    - backward / forward bends
    - lying/ inverted *asanas*
    - *shavasana* (before moving to next regime of *pranayama*.)
    - *pranayama* and meditation session
    - *shavasana*

"Blessed are the flexible for they shall not be bent out of shape.

- Maxim

Asanas

Shavasana
(Corpse pose)

Technique:
- Lie on the back with centre of forehead, chin, navel and pubis in one line.
- Maintain an angle of 45° between the legs.
- Arms on the sides, palms facing upwards.
- Arms should be parallel to legs.
- Close the eyes and consciously relax each and every part of the body, including the mind by auto-suggestion.
- Relate mind and body to yourself and be 'with yourself'.
- Breathe normally with full awareness. Make breathing smooth, soft and effortless and allow mind to descend to heart with each cycle.
- Do not go to sleep during the asana and be fully aware of the breathing and the relaxed state of the body and mind.
- Slowly be aware of all the body parts and open the eyes gently.

Benefits:
- Regulates clean blood supply to the whole body, thus rejuvenating it.
- Reduces physical, mental and emotional stress, strain and fatigue of all kinds.
- Soothes the nerves and the mind.
- Reduces basal metabolic rate, pulse rate and stabilises blood pressure.
- Gives total relaxation to the body; especially recommended after a hard day's work to remove fatigue. Recommended before going to sleep if suffering from insomnia.
- Pacifies anger with regular practice.

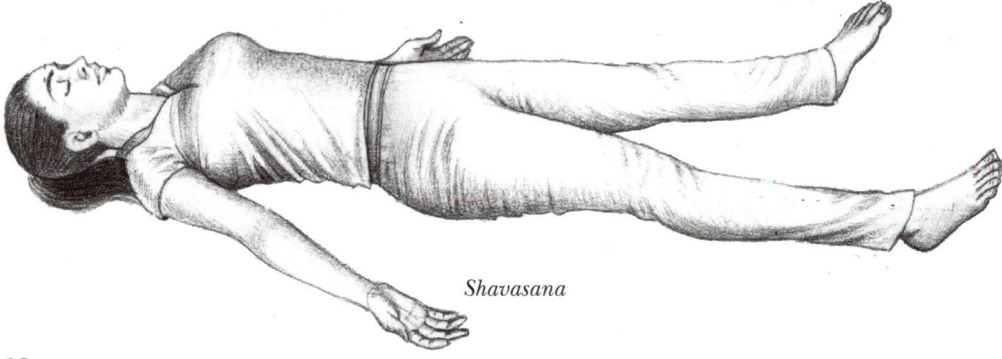
Shavasana

Padmasana
(Lotus pose)

Technique:
- Sit with both feet straight.
- Bend the right knee and place outer border of right foot on the left groin. Similarly the left foot border on the right groin.
- The position of the heels is adjusted so that they are both pressing on the nearest part of the abdomen.
- The palms facing up resting on the knees with index fingers and thumbs in *gyan mudra*.
- Concentrate on Third Eye *Chakra* (medula plexus).
- Keep the head and the spinal column straight, but without straining. Maintain the pose and breathe normally.
- Return to the original position by retracing the steps. Slowly be aware of all the body parts and open the eyes gently.

Benefits:
- Tranquilises the mind and the heart.
- Relieves stiffness from knees and joints.
- Guards against rheumatism.
- Reduces fat around thighs and calves.
- Increases blood flow to the pelvic organs and gonads; this invigorates the coccyx region and the nerves of sacrum.
- Improves digestion.
- Perfect posture for meditation.

Note: In case of difficulty in attaining the said posture, i.e. with both feet on the thighs, 'Half Lotus' pose can be adopted with one foot on the thigh and the other on the ground.

Padmasana

pinkyoga

*Sukhasana**
(Comfortable posture)

Technique:
- Sit with both legs straight.
- Bend the right knee and place its heel on the ground in front of the genital without exerting any pressure.
- Bend the left knee and place the foot in front of the right foot.
- Push a cushion, say 2" (inches) thick, under the buttocks to provide a slight tilt forward.
- Keep the head and spinal column straight, but without straining.
- Place hands on the knees, as in *Padmasana*; maintain *Gyan Mudra* and concentrate on third eye.
- Breathe normally and maintain the pose.

Benefits:
- Identical to those of Lotus posture.
- Ideal for those who find *Padmasana* difficult.
- Less tiring, yet effective.

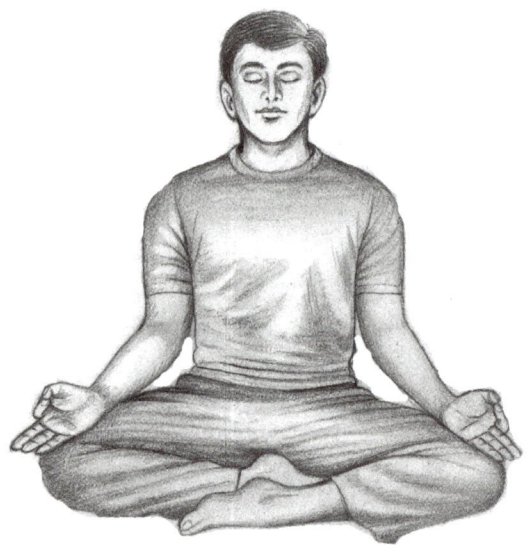

Sukhasana

*Modified

Tadasana
(Stretch Pose)

Technique:
- Lie flat on the back.
- Take both hands over the head, parallel to each other and lock fingers with palms facing outwards.
- Keep legs together.
- Now breathe in and stretch the upper half of the body upwards, whilst lower half being pulled downwards. Hold breath for about 8-10 secs.
- Slowly breathe out and relax the body.
- Repeat 4-6 times.

Benefits:
- Helps in gaining height, particularly in growing children.
- Makes spinal cord attain correct posture; particularly recommended for those with a hump or a hunch.
- Helps in correcting solar plexes.
- Relaxes the body and improves blood circulation.
- Beneficial in backache and cervical spondylitis.
- Relieves sciatica and associated problems.

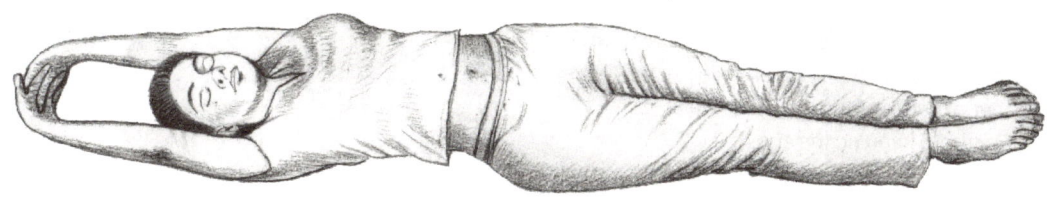

Tadasana

pinkyoga

Surya Namaskar
(Sun Salutation)

Technique:
Surya Namaskar comprises **twelve postures** done contiguously, as described further in different positions. Also there are 12 mantras to be chanted during the positions.

First Position:
- Stand erect; heels together, feet open.
- Fold arms, elbows outward and join hands together in front of the centre of the chest.
- Keep the breathing normal.
- Concentration on the Third Eye *chakra* (*Ajnan chakra* or medula plexus).
- Chant the mantra *'om mitraye namah'*.

Second Position:
- Stretch arms overhead while breathing in keeping them parallel and close to ears.
- Bend backwards slowly as much as possible (without bending the arms).
- Concentrate on throat *chakra* (*vishudha chakra* or carotid plexus).
- Chant the matra *'om ravaye namah'*.

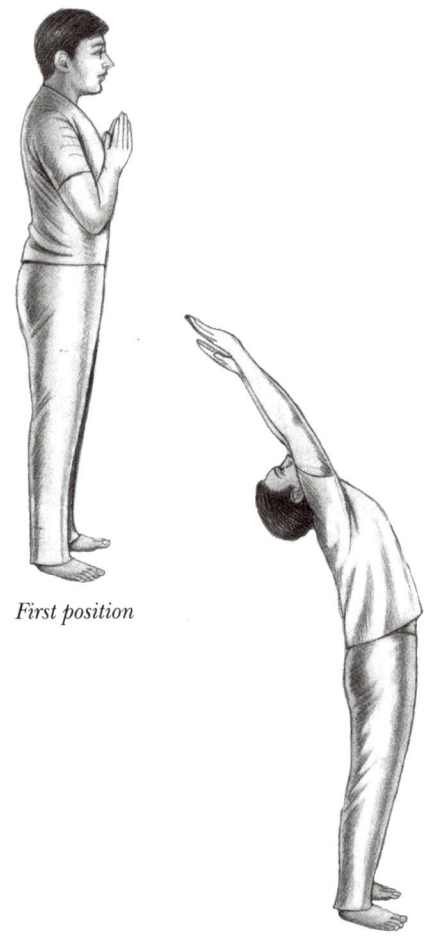

First position

Second position

To Good Health – Sex...Vigour...Vitality

Third Position:
- Slowly bend forward while breathing out.
- Try and touch the ground with fingers and palms (if possible), without exerting unduly.
- Try and touch your knees with your forehead; but make sure there is no undue strain on the back.
- DO NOT bend the knees.
- Concentrate on manipur *chakra* (solar plexus or epigastric plexus).
- Chant the mantra '*om savitre namah*'.

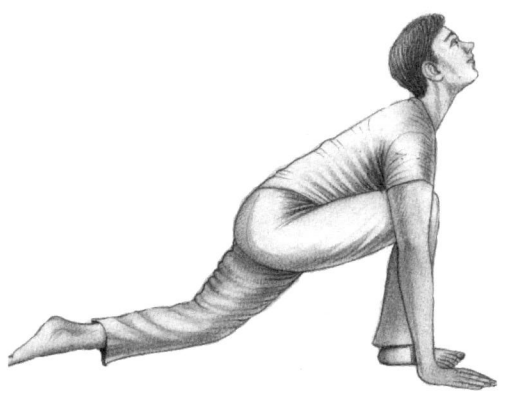

Fourth position

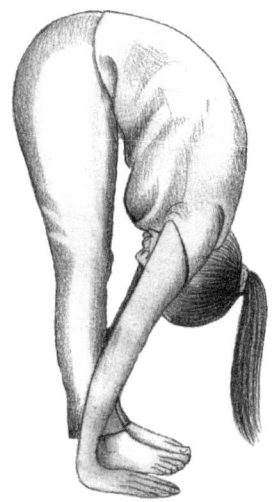

Third position

Fourth Position:
- Breathing in, take the left leg back, stretched on the ground with knee and foot touching the ground. Palms on the ground with fingers together.
- Looking up, push the chest forward back arched appropriately and head backwards; eyes looking towards the sky. Right knee to be placed between the two arms and should be pressing against the chest. Breathe normally.
- Concentrate on '*swadhishthan chakra*' (abdomen *chakra* or hypogastric plexus).
- Chant the mantra '*om pooshney namah*'.

pinkyoga

Fifth Position:
- Raise the hips by straightening the knees; allowing the tail bone to become the highest point (move head, shoulders and chest downwards and backwards, as required).
- Stretch the legs by allowing the heels to touch the ground (slight pull on sciatica may be felt), maintaining the tail bone as the highest point.
- Concentrate on '*Sahastrar Chakra*' (crown *chakra* or the cerebral gland).
- Chant the mantra '*om khagaye namah*'.

Sixth Position:
- Bring slowly the body parallel to ground and lie flat.
- The whole body, i.e. the chin, chest, knees should be touching the ground.
- Lift the hips up slightly and breathe normally in this position.
- Concentrate on '*anahat chakra*' (heart *chakra* or cardiac plexus).
- Chant the mantra '*om bhanave namah*'.

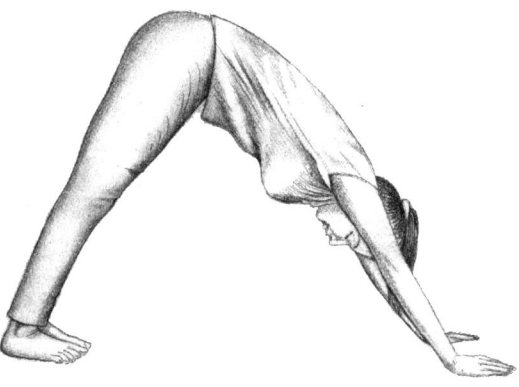

Fifth position

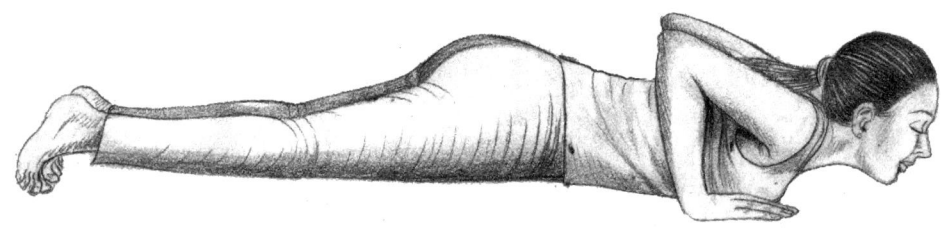

Sixth position

To Good Health – Sex...Vigour...Vitality

Seventh Position:
- Breathing in, raise and extend the head, neck, chest, abdomen, thighs, knees and legs completely by gradually straightening the arms; keep feet about one foot apart.
- Throw the head as back as possible.
- Push chest forward and tighten hip muscles.
- Maintain the pose by resting only on the palms and extended vertical toes. Breathe normally.
- Concentrate on *'mooladhar chakra'* (root *chakra* or pelvic plexus).
- Chant the mantra *'om hiranya garbhaye namah'*.

Eighth Position:
- Switch to the fifth position.
- Chant the mantra *'om suryaye namah'*.

Ninth Position:
- Go back to the fourth position (with right leg behind, this time).
- Chant the mantra *'om adityaye namah'*.

Tenth Position:
- Go to the third position.
- Chant the mantra *'om arkaye namah'*.

Eleventh Position:
- Switch to the second position.
- Chant the mantra *'om marichiye namah'*.

Twelfth Position:
- Come back to the first position.
- Chant the mantra *'om bhaskaraye namah'*.

Benefits:
- Beneficial to all organs from head to toe in the body.
- Invigorates stomach, lungs, liver, kidneys, gall bladder, small and big intestines.
- Strengthens the spine and makes thoracic region supple.
- A complete package that has lots of other benefits.

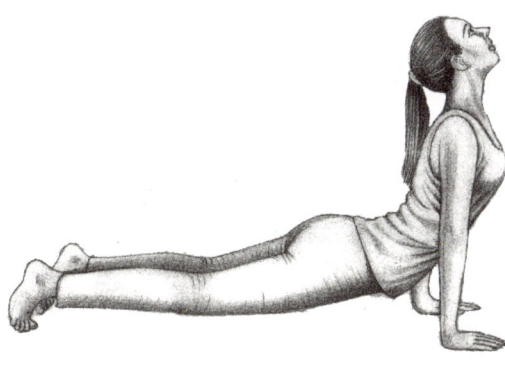

Seventh position

Note: *After Surya Namaskar, shavasana must be practised for 2-3 minutes.*

Vajrasana
(Hero's pose)

Technique:
- Kneel on the knees and fold both legs in such a way that the right (big) toe overlaps the left (big) toe.
- Open the heels as wide as possible so as to make a seat for buttocks to fit in.
- Now slowly sit and rest the buttocks in between the heels. Keep a gap of about 4"- 6" between the knees.
- Keep both the hands on the knees, palms facing down.
- Keep the back erect, look straight and breathe normally.

Benefits:
- Strengthens the spine and removes stiffness from the toes, ankles and knees.
- Reduces fat around the thighs, calves and makes legs shapely.
- More blood flow is directed to the stomach area, which thus improves digestion and cures problems like dyspepsia, flatulence and indigestion.
- Helps to overcome genito-urinary disorders and problems of prostrate, uterus, testes and ovaries.
- Recommended for menstrual disorders: dysmenorrhoea (painful periods).
- Removes fatigue, if practised after a tiring day.
- It boosts the production of white blood corpuscles (WBCs); thus makes robust defence mechanism promoting good health.

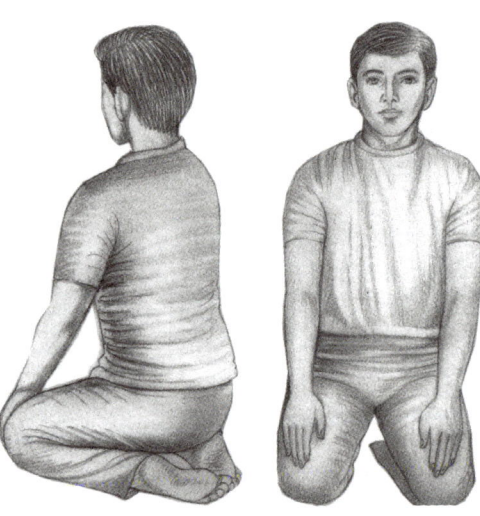

Vajrasana

Note: *It is the only posture which can be practised soon after meals, to help the process of digestion.*

Gomukhasana
(Cow's Face pose)

Technique:
- Sit on the floor, bend right leg at knee and place the right foot horizontally under the hips. Gently sit over it.
- Bend left knee and place the left thigh on top of the right thigh with outer border of left foot resting horizontally on the floor, toes pointing backwards, or **sit in Vajrasana**. Raise left arm, and place palm facing forward between the shoulder blades.
- Take right arm behind, bend it at elbow (facing the ceiling/sky) and place the palm facing backward between the shoulder blades.
- Clasp fingers of both hands and bring the hands closer to each other by allowing both elbows to stretch backwards.
- Keep the back erect. Concentrate on *'anahat chakra'*.
- Maintain the pose and breathe normally.
- Repeat the pose by reversing the positions of arms (and legs if not in *Vajrasana*).

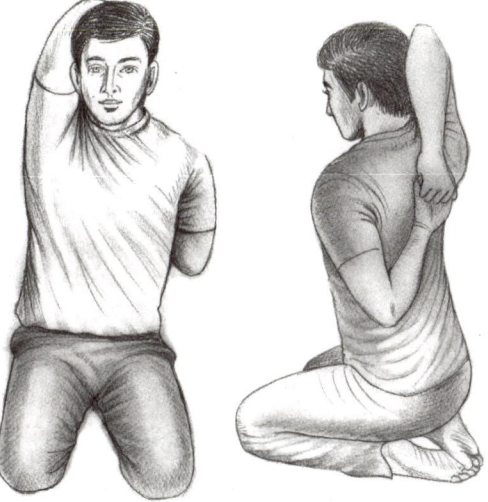

Gomukhasana

Benefits:
- Loosens all small and big joints; recommended for arthritis patients.
- Broadens chest and strengthens heart and lungs.
- Reduces fat around arms, shoulders, thighs and calves and strengthens them.
- Tones gonads; checks undue enlargement of testes.
- Helps to overcome genito-urinary disorders of urinary bladder, and other problems of the uterus and prostate.
- Strengthens the spine.

Supta Vajrasana
(Hero's pose in lying position)

Technique:
- Sit in *Vajrasana*.
- Slowly recline back with one elbow resting on the floor.
- Now rest the second elbow on the floor and extending the arm one at a time, allow the head and the back to rest on the floor.
- Take arms over the head and straighten them or place under the head with one palm on other.
- Maintain the pose and breathe normally. Concentrate on *'manipur chakra'*.
- To return to original position, first hold feet (ankles) and slowly rise.
- Now lean forward and rest in *Shashankasana* (page. 29).

Benefits:
- Reduces congestion in the pelvic organ and loosens ankles, knees, hip and shoulder joints. Beneficial for people suffering from arthritis.
- Tones islets of langerhans, ardrenals and gonads, and benefits people suffering from endocrine disorders like diabetes, and disorders of sexual glands (menstrual).
- Expands chest and lungs and greatly helps to overcome disorders like: asthma, bronchitis and chronic obstructive lung disease.
- Helps to remove postural defects of spine (hump at the back).
- Perfect therapy to overcome indigestion, flatulence and constipation.
- Tones stomach organs, viz. intestines, liver, kidneys, etc.

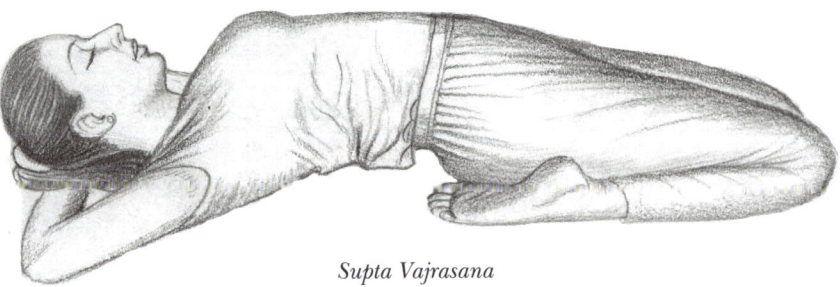

Supta Vajrasana

Shashankasana
(Face down Hero's pose)

Technique:
- Sit in *Vajrasana*.
- Spread the knees a little apart, stretching arms overhead keeping them parallel with palms facing forward, bend trunk and chest forward between them, allowing forehead to rest on the floor.
- Extend the arms forward to rest on the floor. Buttocks should not lift from heels.
- Maintain the pose and breathe normally. Concentrate on '*gyan chakra*' (third eye).
- Inhale and return to the original position.

Benefits:
- This is upasana (reverse posture) of *Supta Vajrasana* and must follow it.
- Improves blood supply to the brain, head and neck.
- Calms the mind and removes mental and physical fatigue.
- Loosens ankles, knee, hip and shoulder joints to soothe arthritis complaints.
- Greatly helps in overcoming:
  - endocrine disorders: diabetes, adrenals and gonads (menstrual).
  - gastro-intestinal disorders: of stomach, liver, spleen, pancreas and intestines.
  - genito-urinary disorders; of urinary bladder, kidneys, uterus, ovaries and testes.
- Stabilises vertebrae on the spine.
- Provides relief in complaints of stool obstruction, constipation, etc.

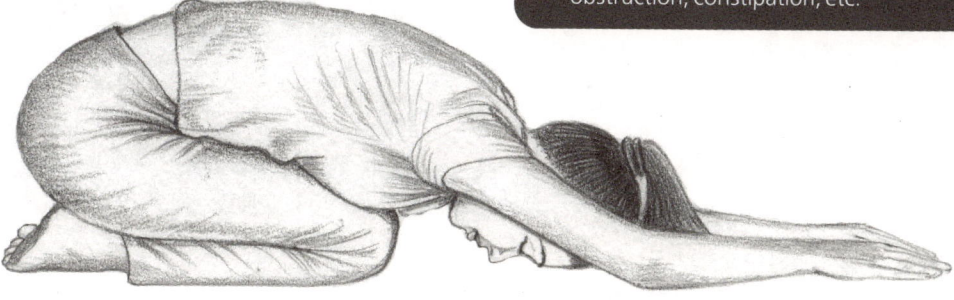

Shashankasana

pinkyoga

Vakrasana
(Spinal Twist pose)

Technique:
- Sit with legs stretched out in the front.
- Bend the right leg, bring it over the left and place the foot flat on the floor just outside the left knee.
- Keep the right hand flat on the floor behind the body and keep the back as straight as possible.
- Now raise the left arm, bring it over the right knee and grasp the right ankle.
- Start exhaling; at the same time begin twisting and turning the waist, chest, neck and head in the direction of the right arm. Twist and turn as much as you comfortably can.
- Hold the breath for 6-8 seconds in this position. At this stage the spine should be straight upwards. Always remember the axis of rotation is the spine and NOT the right arm.
- Then start inhaling slowly and return to the original position by retracing steps.
- Now repeat the *asana* with right leg stretched and left going over.

Benefits:
- Strengthens all organs/glands of waist and abdominal areas, viz. adrenal, kidneys, pancreas, liver (gall-bladder), ovary in females and testicles in males.
- Tones spine and loosens all joints to help overcome arthritis problems.
- Reduces fat around thighs, arms and waist. Tones the lungs and the heart.
- Beneficial for all types of backaches, stiffness of neck, shoulders and spinal disorders.
- Perfect therapy for urinary troubles and diabetes.

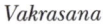

Vakrasana

Bhujangasana
(Cobra pose)

Technique:
- Lie on the belly with forehead touching the floor.
- Bend elbows, bring palms close to shoulders. Elbows should be touching the ground and close to body.
- Keep heels and feet together and pulled outwards.
- Inhale and raise head, neck, chest and upper belly off the floor; with just lower belly, navel and pubis on the floor.
- Extend neck fully backwards (without straining) and brace shoulders backwards. Concentrate on *'visudha chakra'*.
- Keep hips, thighs and knees firm and contracted.
- Hold for 8-10 seconds. Now exhale and return to the original position.
- Repeat 3-5 times.
- Relax with left ear placed on folded arms/hands; palms facing down, on the floor.

Benefits:
- Tones larynx, heart and neck muscles and very useful to overcome problems of cervical and thoracic spondylitis.
- Strengthens complete spine and ideal therapy for high/mid backaches, early slipped discs and sciatica.
- Stimulates thyroid, parathyroid (kidneys), adrenal glands, (pancreas) islets of langerhans.
- Activates pelvic and abdominal organs. Helps to push obstructed stool towards big intestines and rectum; thus relieving constipation.
- Strengthens (in females) ovaries and uterus and helps to regulate menstrual disorders.
- Helps to alleviate voice disorders.

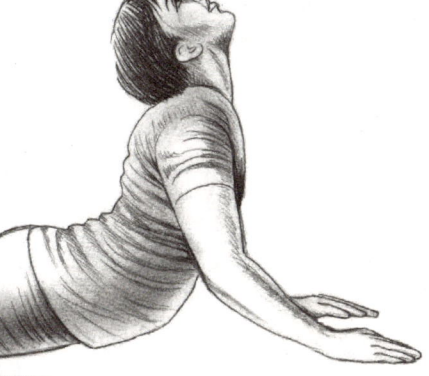

Bhujangasana

pinkyoga

Kandharasana
(Cave Posture)

Technique:
- Lie on the back, fold the knees and bring feet close to buttocks.
- Hold both legs by hands at ankle area.
- Inhale, raise back and buttocks as high as possible; head, shoulders and heels should be on the ground. Hold this position for about 10-15 seconds.
- Exhale, lower the back slowly to the original position.
- Repeat 3-4 times and then relax for a minute in *Shavasana*.

Benefits:
- Stabilises solar plexus.
- Helps to relieve stomach ache and backache.
- Strengthens reproductive (uterus) organs in females.
- In men, useful to overcome sperm problems.
- Tones upper and lower extremity joints in arthritis.
- Boosts blood supply to neck (thyroid/parathyroid) area; useful in respiratory disorders.

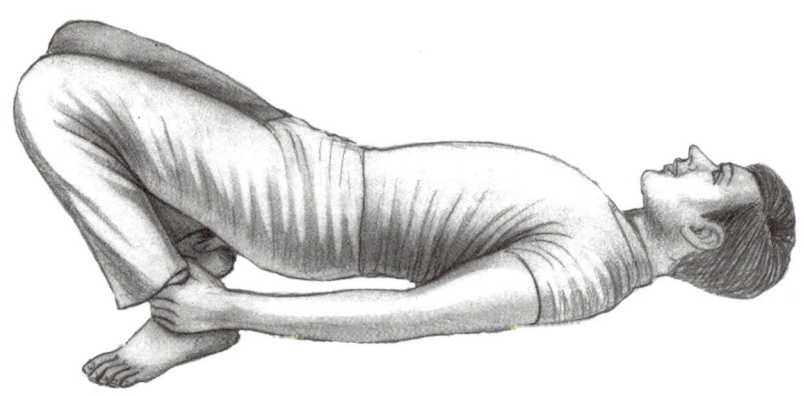

Kandharasana

To Good Health – Sex…Vigour…Vitality

Shalabhasana
(Locust pose)

Technique:
- Lie on the abdomen, clasp the fingers/hands together and place them between the thighs.
- Stretch the chin forward and place it on the ground.
- Inhale, raise the right leg off the ground as high as possible, without bending the knee; hold this position for a few seconds. Exhale and lower the right leg down.
- Inhale and repeat the same with the left leg.
- Now inhale deeply and raise both legs as high as possible. Hold for a few (8-10) seconds and lower them slowly while exhaling.
- Take care to keep the chin pressed to the floor. Concentrate on 'anahat chakra'.
- After completing, relax on the left ear placed on folded arms / hands; palms facing down the floor.

Benefits:
- This is also *Upasana* (counter pose) of *Bhujangasana* and must be performed after it.
- Useful to overcome cervical, thoracic and lumbar spondylitis.
- Helps to relieve upper, mid and low backaches.
- Provides relief in gastro-intestinal disorders of liver, spleen, gall bladder and stomach.
- Tones and stimulates abdominal organs to help cure:
  - Swelling of feet (pedal oedema)
  - Menstrual problems
  - Diabetes, urinary problems and disorders of sex glands
- Helps cure thyroid and parathyroid disorders.
- Tones weak/protruding abdomen.

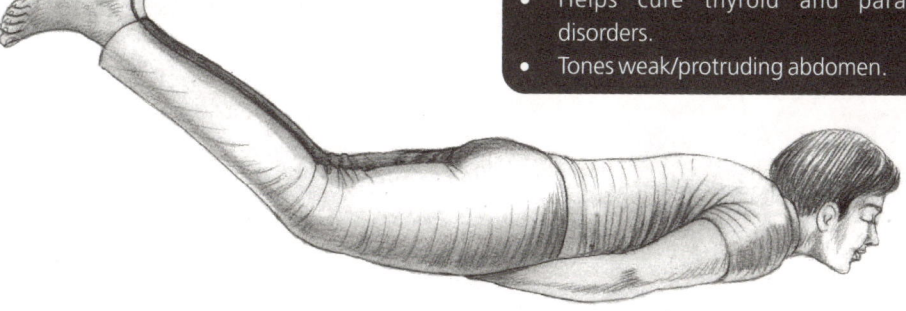

Shalabhasana

Viparitakarani
(Inverted Posture)

Technique:
- Lie on the back and inhale.
- Exhaling, raise legs and hips with the help of arms.
- Bend the arms and hold the hips in the hands so that the body is supported on the elbows, shoulder blades and head.
- The legs should form an angle of 60-70 degrees with the ground.
- Practice abdominal respiration; concentrate on '*visudha chakra*' (carotid plexus).
- Hold as long as comfortable (not more than 5-7 minutes at a time).
- Lower the legs gently to the ground, without lifting the head from the ground.
- Relax in the starting position.

Benefits:
- Abundant blood supply to the neck, throat and head invigorates thyroid / parathyroid, pituitary / pineal glands and nerve centre of the brain.
- Prevents formation of wrinkles on face, pimples and rashes, etc.
- Can cure goiters.
- Sharpens eyesight. Slows the process of hair greying.
- Helps to cure problems of pedal oedema (swelling of feet).

Notes / Precautions:
- *Those suffering from high BP should consult an experienced yoga teacher.*
- *Before performing this asana, one should completely relax.*
- *The advanced postures OF THIS CATEGORY, viz. sarvangasana (shoulder stand) and shirshasan (head stand) ARE ADVISED TO BE PERFORMED ONLY UNDER DIRECT SUPERVISION OF A TEACHER.*

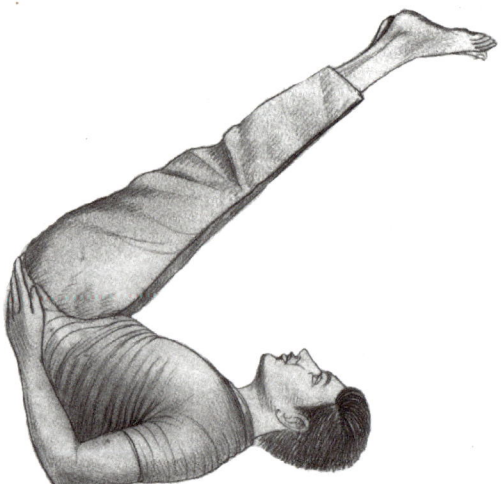

Viparitakarani

Matsyasana*
(Fish Pose)

Technique:
- Lie on the back, legs and feet together.
- Slide the stretched arms under the body so that the hands are under the buttocks (palms facing down).
- Now push the body slightly towards legs; lift torso with the help of elbows and arch the back to lower the head, neck and back, till crown of the head rests on the floor.
- Make sure the load is on the elbows and not on the crown.
- Inhale, pull neck inside as mush as possible and stretch legs; hold for a few seconds. Concentrate on '*gyan chakra*'.
- Now shifting the arms out; lift the upper body up, rest on elbows and look at the feet.
- Then turn the neck left-right-left a few times and rotate clockwise and anti-clockwise; slowly switch to *Shavasana* posture for about 1-2 minutes.
- Repeat 2-4 rounds only.

Benefits:
- This is '*Upasana*' (counter pose) to inverted postures, e.g. '*Viparitakarani, Sarvangasana* and *Shirshasana*' and must be performed after these.
- Good therapy for respiratory disorders, like asthma and bronchitis.
- Activates pituitary, thyroid / parathyroid and overall body balance.
- Eases stiffness of upper extremities, relieves frozen shoulder, cervical and thoracic spondylitis complaints.
- Strengthens neck, lungs, heart and spine.
- Prevents wrinkles on face.
- Tones the stomach and the back muscles and activates the digestive system.
- Gives relief in menstrual disorders.

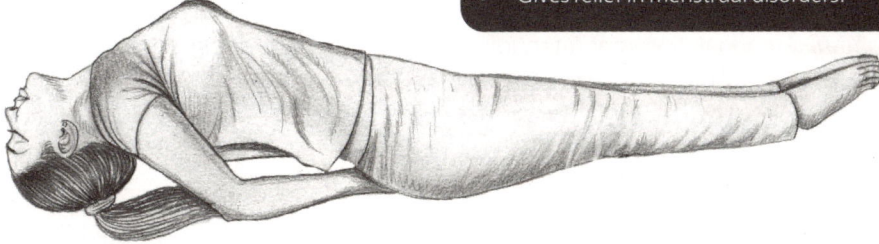

Matsyasana

*Modified

PRANAYAMA

Pranayama – Breath Control

'Breath is spirit. The act of breathing is living.'
- Ancient Yoga Proverb

The Sanskrit word *prana* means 'vital force' (or *chetana*). It also signifies life or breath. '*Ayam*' means the extending of *prana*. In actual context, it means control/management. Hence, *Pranayama* means control of the vital force by concentration and regulated breathing.

Pranayama involves three breathing activities:

- *Purak* (inhalation): The process of breathing in and the passage of air to the lungs through nasal cavities.

- *Rechak* (exhalation): The process of breathing out.

- *Kumbhak* (retention of breath): The process of holding the breath. It could be at two levels, i.e. *antarik kumbhak* (internal retention); holding the breath after inhalation. And *bahya kumbhak* (external retention) is to hold the breath after exhalation.

In our body there are three main *nadis* (channels):

- **Ida Nadi:** This is also referred to as the *moon nadi* or cold and is activated by breathing through the left nostril.

- **Pingala Nadi:** This is a hot one producing heat in the body, also known as *sun nadi* and is activated by breathing through the right nostril.

- **Sushumna Nadi:** This is central or neutral passing through the spine vertebrae from *visudha* to *mooladhar chakra*. Then it gets split into two pathways through both legs; also referred to as sciatica.

The combination of these three could also be understood as positive, negative and earth wires of any electric circuitary. It could well be assumed that bio-electricity is managed in the body through these.

Types of *Pranayama*

The old Yogic texts/scriptures mention upto 50 varieties of *Pranayama*. However, here we would elaborate only five types:

 I. *Anulom Vilom / Nadi Shodhan*
 II. *Ujjayi*
 III. *Kapalbhati*
 IV. *Naad Yoga*
 V. *Yoga Nidra**

[*The *Yoga Nidra* (yogic sleep) has been included herein for two reasons: one for complete relaxation after yoga session, and secondly to synergise the conscious and the subconscious mind, and stronger attunement with self.]

Anulom Vilom / Nadi Shodhan
(Alternate Breathing)

Technique:
- Sit in *Padmasana* or *Sukhasana* (or sit on a chair with back erect).
- Keep spine absolutely straight and relax your thoughts. Left hand should be placed on the knee in *gyan mudra*.
- Place the index finger of right hand on third eye (between eyebrows) and close the right nostril, with the thumb.
- The other three fingers of right hand, i.e. middle, ring and little finger are in folded condition.
- Breathe in through the left nostril briskly.
- Close the left nostril with the curved pad of the three fingers and open the right nostril. Start exhaling slowly and at a leisurely pace. Feel the slow passage of air on your lips.
- After complete exhalation, press the stomach slightly in to push the remaining air volume out of the lungs.
- Now, breathe in briskly through the right nostril and close it with the thumb after inhalation.
- The exhalation, this time, should be slow and leisurely from the left nostril.

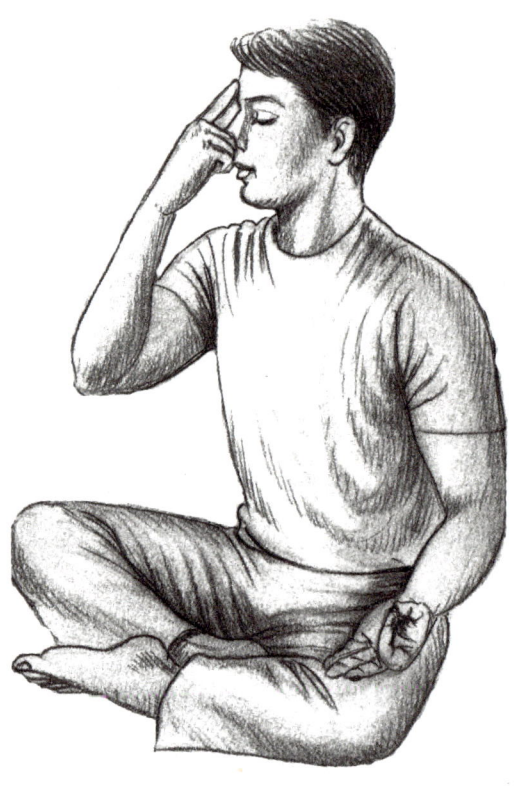

Anulom Vilom / Nadi Shodhan

- This is one cycle. Remember this *Pranayama* has to be done in cycles. Start with 2-3 minutes and gradually you may practice for 10-15 minutes.
- Time proportion initially of inhalation, exhalation is to be maintained the same. But after few weeks of practice and if not suffering from conditions like blood pressure or weak heart or asthma or other lung problems, *kumbhaka* (retention) may be introduced between every inhalation / exhalation.
- The time proportion of *puraka*, *rechaka* and *kumbhaka* should be 1 : 2 : 2 usually. But it can be taken upto 1: 4 : 2 with practice.
- Keep the left hand in *gyan mudra* and concentrate on the *anahat chakra*.
- Remember ONCE THE PROPORTION IS 1 : 2 : 2 or 1 : 4 : 2, THIS *PRANAYAMA* IS CALLED *NADI SHODHAN*, i.e. Purification of *nadis*/channels of *prana*.

Benefits:
- One of the most important *Pranayama* to establish equilibrium of the positive and negative currents bringing life to the body, i.e. balancing bio-electricity.
- Calms and purifies the nerves.
- Helps stabilise the mind and mental faculties.
- Improves the immune system and helps overcome:
  - respiratory disorders: asthma, bronchitis etc. (without *kumbhaka*).
  - stress related disorders peptic ulcers, diabetes, and colitis.
  - cardiovascular disorders: hypertension, angina pectoris (without *Kumbhaka*).
- Recommended to get over insomnia, improve memory and concentration (without *kumbhaka*).
- Helpful in convalescence from various diseases.
- To get over physical or mental fatigue.
- An all-pervasive *Pranayama* to balance all three humors (*vaat*, *pitta* and *kapha*) in the body and usher overall health.

Ujjayi

Technique:
- Sit in *Padmasana/Sukhasana* (or on a chair).
- Keep both hands in *gyana mudra*.
- Turn the tip of the tongue and touch the palate as far back as possible.
- Lower the chin slightly to the sternum.
- Now take long deep breath with snoring sound (from the throat not nasal area).
- Then, exhale slowly without any snoring sound.
- The breathing should be slow and rhythmic.
- Repeat 8-10 cycles.
- Concentrate on '*visudha chakra*'.

Benefits:
- Helps to cure mental disorders like epilepsy, etc.
- Great therapeutic *pranayama* to cure throat infections, tonsillitis, soreness, normal cough and cold complaints.
- Strengthens thyroid and parathyroid glands and wards off nose and ear infections.
- Makes the voice sweet. Recommended specially for singers.
- Helps to overcome snoring disorders and stammering complaints.
- Relieves mental stress and problems of insomnia, depression etc.

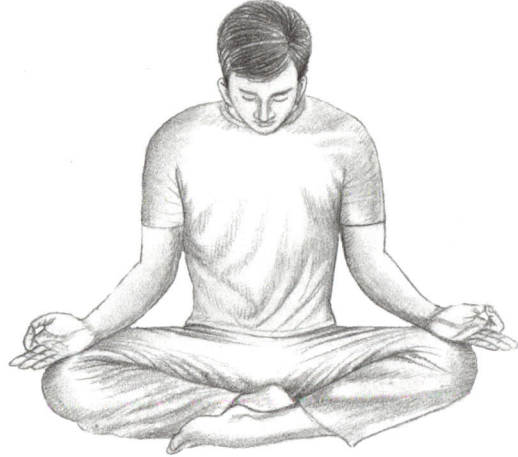

Ujjayi

Kapalbhati

Technique:
- Sit in *Padmasana/Sukhasana* (or on a chair).
- Keep the hands in *gyana mudra*.
- In this *pranayama* the stress is on *rechaka* (exhalation).
- Do *puraka* and carry out *rechaka* in jerks by contracting abdominal muscles around the solar plexus. NO INTENTIONAL BREATHING IN TO BE DONE; HOWEVER SMALL AMOUNTS OF AIR MAY BE ALLOWED TO FLOW IN.
- The frequency initially should be one jerk per second; which could be higher after a few weeks, to two jerks per second.
- Once the full breath is out; relax for a few seconds and start again with fresh *puraka* followed by *rechaka* in jerks.
- Concentrate on *ajneya chakra* (medula plexus).
- Do for 3-5 minutes. (Relax in between if there is back pain or a tired feeling).

Alternative *Kapalbhati*

There is an alternative method to perform *Kapalbhati* – though not commonly practised – considered to be original by some schools of thought.

In this method the neck moves in a rhythmic manner back-to-forth while doing *rechak* and the process is confined to above diaphragm / neck area only. Rest of the body below should remain still.

Benefits:
- Literally *Kapalbhati* translates to *kapal* (skull) and *bhati* (shine), i.e. to shine the skull.
- Relieves and soothes mental nerves and helps cure headache.
- Helps to overcome obesity, dyspepsia, flatulence and problems of liver, gall bladder, kidneys and prostrate glands.
- Cures diseases of phlegm, respiratory tract, allergies, sinusitis, etc.
- Constipation can be cured with regular practice of 3-5 minutes.
- Helps to contain diabetes.
- Strengthens lungs and regular practice helps to unclog arterial blockages. Strengthens weak intestines.
- Clears the toxins from the body and in the process cleanses nasal cavities from bacteria and viruses.

Naad Yoga

Technique:
- Sit in *Padmasana/Sukhasana* (or on a chair).
- Keep hands on the knees in *gyana mudra*.
- Keep back straight; eyes tightly closed and face relaxed.
- Take one or two deep breaths.
- Now take a deep breath and chant OM (*O-U-M*) split in three parts, while slowly and rhythmically exhaling. The time proportion for *O-U-M* for the duration of breath is 1:1:2.
- During this cycle also imagine, upward movement of energy, say in light form, from '*mooladhar*' to '*sashastra*' *chakra*, passing through the *chakras* via the '*sushumna nadi*'.

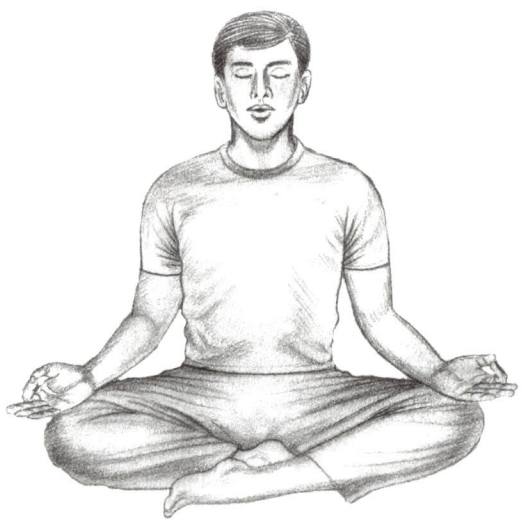

Naad Yoga

Benefits:
- Soothes the entire neurological network and relaxes the mind and the body.
- Ushers in harmony of mind, body and soul.
- Activates *ajneya chakra*; sharpens brain and improves memory.
- The vibrations/reverberations activate the *chakras* – the energy centres – and the latent energy serpent (*kundalini*) at *mooladhar* traverses upwards.

Note: *Detailed activation of 'kundalini' should only be done under guidance of your guru / teacher - as its uncontrolled awakening can spell disastrous effects.*

YOGA NIDRA: YOGIC SLEEP

A calm mind is not disturbed by the waves of thoughts
- **Remez Sasson**

Lie down in *shavasana*.

Take about 10-20 deep breaths and completely relax while slowly letting limbs go loose.

Now take deep breaths again. With every breath you exhale, mentally command your body to 'relax'. Continue for 3-5 minutes.

Focus on each part of the body in the following sequence: 'back, back of the head, top of the head, forehead, right eyebrow, left eyebrow, right eye, left eye, middle of the eyebrow, right cheek, left cheek, right nostril, left nostril, upper lip, lower lip, chin, neck, chest, stomach, and abdomen', without any movement.

Thereafter focus on the 'right hand thumb, index finger, middle finger, ring finger, little finger, palm, wrist, elbow, shoulder, armpit, hip, thigh, knee, calf, heel, sole, the big toe, second toe, third toe, fourth toe, and the fifth.'

Repeat with the left.

Make a positive resolve to yourself. Remind yourself and keep saying: 'I am healthy and happy' or 'I am at complete peace' or 'I am free of all stresses / diseases'. Repeat it everyday.

pinkyoga

Now imagine you are standing in front of a very picturesque place such as a waterfall, a calm beach or a garden full of beautiful and blossomed flowers. Now try and capture every positive detail of the scenery (e.g., clear falling water, abundance of greenery, setting sun, drops of dew on a petal, different colours of flowers, etc.).

Repeat your resolution again 3 times keeping the picturesque scenes in mind. You may go off to sleep after the exercise or else open your eyes, stretch the body and sit up.

BANDHS (Air Locks)

Bandhs are simple yet very effective means to charge, stimulate and strengthen the internal organs in and around our *chakras*. These are:
   Jalandhara Bandh (throat area).
   Uddiyana Bandh (diaphragm area).
   Moola Bandh (root area).

{ **NOTE:** *The* bandhs *can be performed in both conditions of either* aantarika kumbhaka *(fully inhaled) or* bahya kumbhak *(fully exhaled) position.* }

Jalandhara Bandh

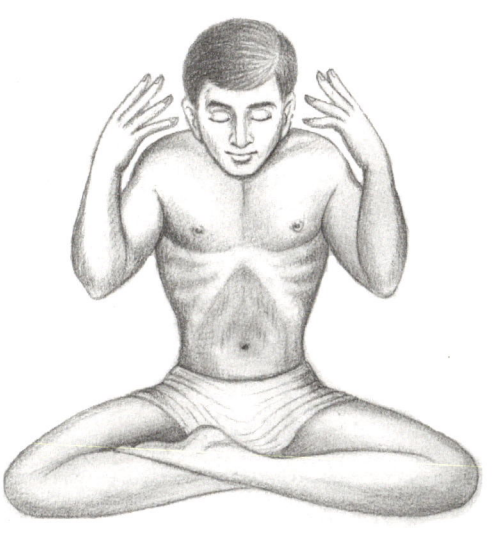

Jalandhara Bandh

Technique:
- Sit in *Padmasana/Sukhasana* (or on a chair with back erect).
- Put aantarik/ bahya kumbhak.
- Lower the chin to the sternum.
- Keep the chest out, back erect.
- Eyes closed or half closed focused at the middle of eyebrows.
- Hold breath till comfortably tolerable, then, release slowly and take a few deep breaths.
- Repeat a few times.

Benefits:
- Strengthens thyroid / parathyroid glands.
- Makes voice sweet.
- Avoids double chin formation.
- Beneficial in throat disorders.
- Awakens *visudha chakra* (throat *chakra*).
- Due to locking of *Ida*, *Pingala*, the *Prana* starts flowing through *Sushumna*.

pinkyoga

Uddiyana Bandh

Technique:
- Sit in *padmasana / sukhasana* or even standing position with body bent forward, hands placed on knees.
- Perform *aantarik / bahya kumbhak*.
- Pull belly inwards (towards back) as far as possible.
- Hold till comfortable, then release slowly and take a few deep breaths.
- Repeat a few times.

Benefits:
- Awakens *manipur chakra* (solar plexus).
- Helps cure digestion disorders.
- Massages stomach organs and diaphragm area.
- Helps reduce fat around the waist.
- Rejuvenates digestion, has preventive/curative effects on problems like constipation, dyspepsia, etc.

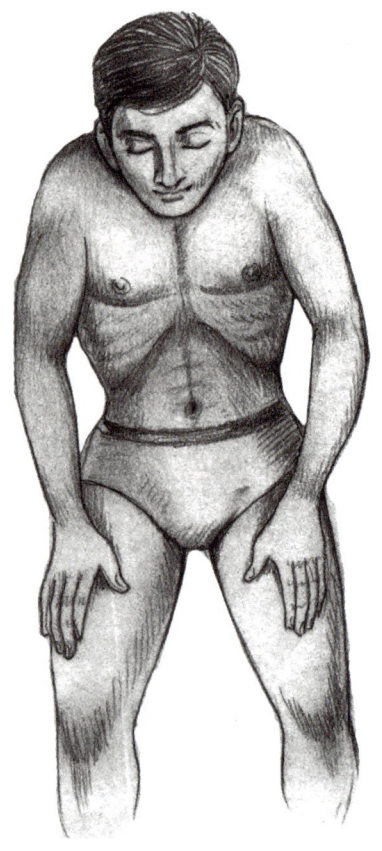

Uddiyna Bandh

To Good Health – Sex...Vigour...Vitality

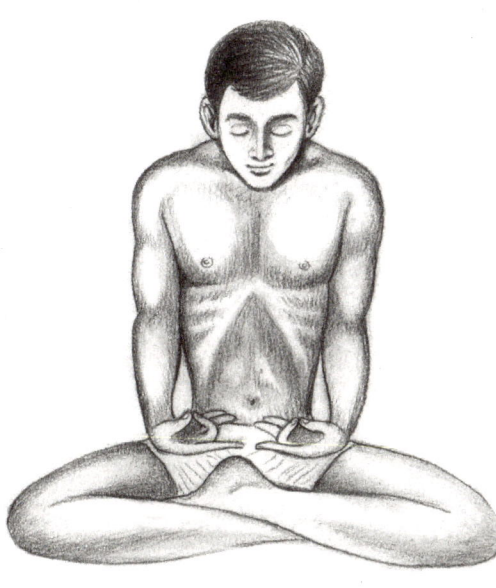

Moola Bandh

Benefits:
- Awakenes *mooladhar chakra*.
- Makes *kundalini* upward moving.
- Helps cure problems of indigestion and diseases like piles, constipation, etc.
- Strengthens spermatozoa and helps to overcome sterility.

Maha Bandh

Technique:
- All *bandhs* performed together.

Benefits:
- *Prana* moves upwards.
- Spermatozoa strengthens; improves vigour.
- With this *Ida*, *Pingala*, and *Sushumna* share proper bio-energy movements like +ve, -ve, and neutral current flow.

Moola Bandh

Technique:
- Sit in *padmasana* / *sukhasana* or on a chair with back erect.
- Perform *kumbhaka*.
- Pull upwards the anus and urogenital organ.
- Hold the breath till comfortable, then release slowly and take a few deep breaths.
- Repeat a few times.

MEDITATION

'If you want to find God, hang out in the space between your thoughts'
- **Alan Cohen**

The human evolution takes place on three different planes: mental, physical and spiritual.

The purity, serenity by virtue of *yama*, *niyama*, *asanas* and *pranayama* provides a soothing backdrop to the 'self'. The atonement then is almost effortless in case of senses / perceptions (*indriyas*) and makes them 'inward' bound that slowly and steadily establishes equilibrium (of mind-body).

The condition of practitioner is more or less like – eyes are open but does not see externally, ears do not hear, and hands and limbs do not move. The external sensory existence almost ceases and the *indriyas* are looking 'inward' from worldly matters.

[**CAUTION:** The practitioner is advised to proceed to the three stages of '*dharana-dhyan-samadhi*' under the guidance of one can say a guru / teacher because these are the final stages of connecting the self to the cosmos or say *atma* to *parmatma* and energy upheavals could have adverse effects.]

Dharana: Dhyan: Samadhi

Dharana is concentration. It is focusing the mind on something within – e.g., heart, third eye, nose tip – or outside the body, e.g. a deity or a primordial sound given by the teacher / guru.

Dhyana (meditation) is the unbroken flow of thoughts towards the object of concentration. It can be called 'prolonged concentration'.

When the mind can be made to flow uninterruptedly towards the same object for 12 seconds, one is said to have learnt the process of concentration. If concentration continues for 2 minutes and 24 seconds, one is said to be practising meditation. If the same continues for 12 minutes and 24 seconds, it is a state of lower *samadhi*. And if this state of lower *samadhi* can be maintained for 5 hours, 45 minutes and 36 seconds, one is said to be in (*nirvikalpa*) *samadhi*.

Samadhi (or absorption) is a state when the object of concentration and the mind of the perceiver becomes one. When concentration, meditation and *samadhi* are brought to bear upon one subject, it is called *samyam*.

During meditation the object of concentration may change in form, time and rhythm. The whole process of meditation therefore varies from person to person and day to day.

The *indriya*-centric meditation techniques, their detailed learning and practice; the guidance from a guru / teacher must be solicited. Two simple techniques, viz. vibration meditation and movement meditation are discussed in the following chapters.

Vibration Meditation

This method of meditation involves the use of auspicious sounds / syllables (e.g. OM) for releasing stress.

- Sit in *Padmasana/Sukhasana* or lie down in *shavasana*.

- Relax the body completely by taking a few deep breaths and letting limbs loose.

- Select a word/phrase/*mantra*, the chanting of which makes you feel good. The chosen word/*mantra* could range from a single positive word like 'love', 'peace', 'harmony' or say the Gayatri mantra or any other sound one wishes to recite.

- Repeatedly chant it and focus on the vibrations through your body.

- Feel the vibrations from the top of your body to the hands and feet (tip to toe). Some have the tendency to clench their muscles when they are tense. It is important that you roll the sound through your body so that you can clear out the tightness in your muscles.

- Keep repeating it till a meditative state of relaxation is attained.

MOVEMENT MEDITATION

This meditation involves soft, rhythmic, gentle flowing movements to create a meditative state. Such movements help to derive energy from the earth while releasing stress from the body, thus relaxing the mind.

- Switch on the music of your choice

- Stand in an area with adequate free space around you.

- Take a few deep breaths and relax the body

- Concentrate by visualising your feet connected to the earth, drawing energy from the earth

- Gradually sway your body with the sound of the music. Dance if you like

- Focus your attention on the movement and on the vibration of the sound

- Allow yourself to get absorbed in the rhythm of movements and the beauty of your body as it moves. Feel the music flow through from *mooladhar* to *sahastrar chakra* as if striking the notes *sa, re, ga, ma, pa, dha, ni . . . sa.*

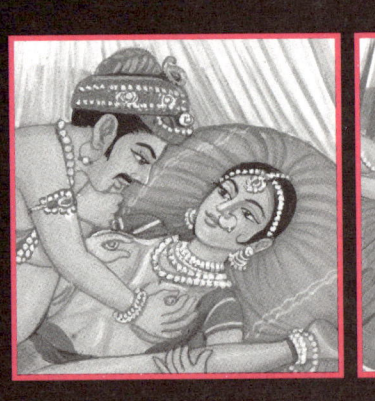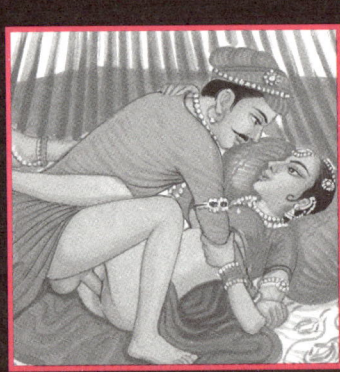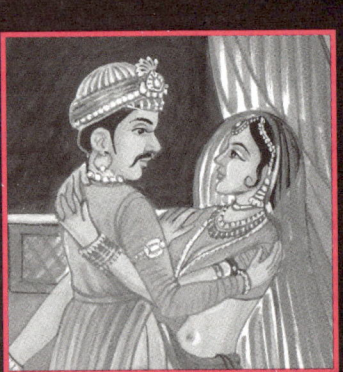

Kamasutric Art of Love

'Sex is Emotion in Motion'

- Mae West

KAMASUTRIC ART OF LOVE

According to the Hindu philosophy, the life on earth passes through the acquisition of three stages, i.e. *dharma*, *artha* and *kama*, one or the other element acquiring more importance through different *ashrams* (phases) of life, presumed to be hundred years.

Dharma (religion) should be learnt from the holy scriptures or from those conversant.

Arth (wealth) the acquisition of land, gold, wealth, etc., should be learnt from those conversant with commerce.

Kama (lovemaking) is the art of enjoyment by the five senses of seeing, smelling, hearing, tasting, and touching assisted by the mind together with the soul. The embodiment of mind, body and soul activation should ideally be learnt from *Kamasutra* (aphorisms on love).

Sage Vatsyayana composed *Kamasutra* from the percepts of the Holy Writ, while leading the life of a religious student wholly engaged in the contemplation of the deity. Vatsyayana in his own way was thus bestowed with apt congruence of divinity (energy) and material existence (matter). Therefore, it is considered that a prudent person should attend to *dharma*, *artha* and *kama*, obtain success in everything undertaken, without becoming slave of one's passion.

It is said 'Truth is Beauty, Beauty is Truth' because beauty can transport the mind into meditative zone, instantly.

In Eastern and Central India, places like Konark and Khajuraho, there are sculptures depicting erogenous postures of male / female congress on temples linking it to divinity and there are explanations / opinions of different schools of thoughts towards it, like:

- A man and a woman in embrace typify the ultimate union of the soul with the Divine.

- These erotic postures save the temples from being struck by the lightning – maybe due to high energy levels of the union.

- A mythological logic given is that the God of rain and thunder, Indra, himself a great connoisseur of *kama*, would not damage anything related to it.

- Another theory is that erogenous sculptures on temple walls were meant to test whether the devotee had purged his mind of worldly thoughts before entering the temple.

- Yet another Hindu sect considers *yoga* (spiritual exercise) and *bhoga* (physical pleasure) as two different paths leading to the same goal that is *moksha*, self deliverance. According to these sects, enjoyment of sex can help one transcend into a *samadhi,* and thereby attain *nirvana* (salvation).

- A verse from *Brihadaranyaka* Upanishad (4-3-2) corroborates: 'That indeed in his form which transcends desires, is bereft of merits and demerits, and is fearless. As a man fully embraced by his dear wife knows nothing external or internal, even so this infinite entity fully embraced by the Supreme Self knows nothing external or internal. That indeed is his form in which all objects of desire have been realised, in which they have become the self, and which is devoid of desire and beyond grief'.

To Good Health - Sex...Vigour...Vitality

- As per sexologists, presumably the releases of energy through the congress burns the body's calories to the tune of 115-220 kcals. The congress also triggers production of an anti-depressant chemical *Dopamin* in the brain, an explanation to relaxation, post-facto.

Kama and theories of *kama* should **always** be understood / learnt in a professional manner. The book describes concisely the 'relevants' as regards to *kama* for the contemporary society, and particularly for education of new entrants to *Grahastha Ashrama*. These are:-

Classification

The classification of male / female species is based on length of the *lingam* (male genital) and depth of the *yoni* (female genital).

Male	Lingam on Erection
Shash (Hare-Man)	About 3 inches
Vrishabha (Bull-Man)	About 4.5 inches
Ashira (Horse-Man)	About 6 inches

Female	Depth of *Yoni*
Mrigi (deer woman)	About 3 inches
Ashwini (Mare-Woman)	About 4.5 inches
Karini (Elephant-Woman)	About 6 inches

> **NOTE:** *These yonis may be of four types - the best is whose surface inside is soft like lotus petals, the other has some flashy knots / rises, and then the ones with corrugated surface and not that enjoyable. The worst, of course, are those which have the inside surface very rough.*

Ideal and properly enjoyable congress works out when compatibility proportions of male / female are properly meted out.

External Enjoyments

These are the processes that should always precede internal enjoyments or coition. Broadly these may be categorised as under:

- *Aalinganas* (Embraces)

- *Chumban* (Kisses)

- *Nakhadana* (Unguiculations): Use of nails, with moderate pressure

- *Dashanas* (Morsications): Use of teeth with carefully applied pressure

- *Keshagrahanas* (Manipulating the hair)

Herein, the kisses may need brief elaboration; others are expected to spring-up quite naturally during the foreplay period.

The intensity of kisses and form can differ depending upon the time of separation, the frame of mind or mood during foreplay, etc. of the partners. Most commonly it can be either spouse taking upper or lower lip at a time. One can also be tempted for both lips and mouth to be taken or the inside of mouth. Sometimes mood changer can be a forced kiss till the other partner gives in.

Internal Enjoyments

Kamasanas

Kamasanas is the art of male / female congress, after the external enjoyments. It is during this *asana* that actual insertion / penetration of *lingam* into the *yoni* is executed.

These *Kamasutric asanas* have benefits too besides providing variety and pleasure, such as:

(i) Almost all extremities / joints are exercised.

(ii) Partial release of *Kundalini* upwards.

(iii) Release of endorphin and dopamin chemicals giving pleasure, relaxation to the neurological systems.

[**Caution:** Herein, one must take precaution if suffering from orthopaedic or any other serious problem. Just to quote an example if a person is suffering from cervical spondylitis he / she must choose a comfortable posture (as explained below), variations and should not bend forward.]

There are five main / generic asanas (postures) of congress with subdivisions too. Some selective stimulating postures are discussed hereafter.

A) *Uttana-Bandha* (Supine posture): Under this generic one, four shall be elaborated i.e. 'Aa', 'Abl', 'Ac', 'Ad'.

B) *Tiryak* (Aslant posture): Shall have two sub divisions 'Ba', 'Bb'.

C) *Upavishta* (Sitting posture): Here we would discuss two varieties i.e. 'Ca', 'Cb'..

D) *Utthita* (Standing posture): This would have two varieties i.e. 'Da', 'Db'.

E) *Vyanta-Bandha* (Lying posture): Has two varieties; 'Ea', 'Eb'

F) *Purushayita-Bandh* (Supine with man lying on the back): Under this two varieties are explained, 'Fa', 'Fb'.

A. *Uttana Bandha*

In this generic *asana,* the woman is in supine position. The four subdivisions of the same are discussed as follows:

Aa. *Sampada-Uttana-Bandha*
- Partner (woman) in supine posture, that is lying on her back with face up.
- Both her legs raised and placed on the partner's shoulders.
- Man sits close to her upon his hams and enjoys her after insertion.

Ab. *Nagara-Uttana-Bandha (Plate 1)*
- Partner (woman) in supine posture that is lying on her back with face upwards.
- Both her legs raised and placed on either side of husband's waist.
- Man sits between her legs and enjoys after penetration.

Ac. *Traivikrama-Uttana-Bandha*
- Partner (woman) in supine posture, that is lying on her back with face upwards.
- Her one leg rests on the carpet / bed.

- The other leg is placed on the man's head.
- Man supporting himself on his both hands, enjoys after insertion.

Ad. *Vyompada-Uttana-Bandha* (Plate 2)
- Partner (woman) in supine posture that is lying on her back with face upwards.
- Woman raises both her legs with both hands as far back as her hair.
- Man sitting close to her with both hands upon her breasts.

B. Tiryaka

The essence of this generic asana is that the woman lies on her side. The other two subdivisions include:

Ba. *Samputa-Tiryaka-Bandha*
- Both partners lying on their sides.
- Legs straight, without any shift.
- Enjoy after penetration.

Bb. *Karkata-Tiryak-Bandh* (Plate 3)
- Both partners lying on their sides.
- Man then moves in between woman's thighs.
- One thigh under him, the other over his flanks, a little below the breast and enjoys.

C. *Upavishta* (Sitting Posture)

The subdivisions under this category include the following:

Ca. *Padmasana* (Plate 4)
- Man sits cross-legged on the bed/carpet.
- Takes woman on the lap, with both hands on her shoulders. And enjoys her after slow insertion.

Cb. *Yugmapada-Asana*
- Man sits with both legs wide apart.
- Executes insertion / penetration and then presses woman's thighs together and enjoys her.

D. *Utthita*

This category of standing posture has two subdivisions highlighted.

Da. *Janu-Kuru-Utthitha-Bandh*
- Both man and woman stand facing each other.
- Man then lifts the woman, passing his arms under her knees and supporting them on his inner elbows.
- Woman is posited as high as his waist and the partner enjoys after penetration. Woman clasps his neck with both hands.

Db. *Hari-Vikrama-Utthita-Bandh* (Plate 5)
- Both man and woman stand facing each other.
- Man raises one leg of the woman, the other leg is in standing position.
- Partners enjoy each other after insertion.

E. *Vyanta-Bandh*

In this generic posture the woman lies on her stomach i.e. prone, with breasts and stomach to the bed / carpet. Two selective subdivisions include:

Ea. *Denuka-Vyanta-Bandh [Cow Posture] (Plate 6)*
- In this posture, the woman places herself on all fours, supporting on her hands and feet (not knees).
- The man approaches from behind and enjoys like a bull by falling on her and holding her from the waist.

Eb. *Aybha-Vyanta-Bandh [Elephant posture]*
- Woman lies down with face, breasts, stomach and thighs touching the bed / carpet.
- Man extends himself upon her and sitting like an elephant, i.e. bending with the small of the back, effects insertion and enjoys.

F. *Purushayita Bandh*

In this *asana*, the man is in supine position, i.e. lying on the back with face upwards. This form has two popular subdivisions:

Fa. *Viparita-Bandh (Plate 7)*
- Man in supine position on the bed/carpet.
- Woman lying on his outstretched body with breasts touching his bosom.
- Woman presses his waist with her hands, facilitates insertion and moves her hips in various directions and both partners enjoy.

pinkyoga

Fb. *Purushayita-Bharamara Bandh:*
- Man in supine position upon bed/carpet.
- Woman squats on man's thighs.
- After insertion she closes her legs firmly and enjoys the movements, thereafter.

A few guidelines to be always kept in mind :

- The place for congress should be dimly lit, well-ventilated and not cluttered.

- The external enjoyments / foreplay should be sombre initially and carried on till woman is amorous.

- *Moolabandh* can be practised intermittently to prolong the joy of orgasm, particularly towards the final stages.

- In between 'electric-*pranayama*', i.e. breathing in through the nose and slowly breathing out through the mouth with lips in circular mode like when whistling, enhances the stamina.

- Electric-*pranayama* (5-8 breaths) should be necessarily done at the end of congress.

- Proper cleaning should be done at the end, preferably with warm water. Male partner must urinate after the congress.

- *Vajrasana* should be done for almost 3-4 mins; before settling to sleep or work.

- A glass of milk after the congress rejuvenates the body completely.

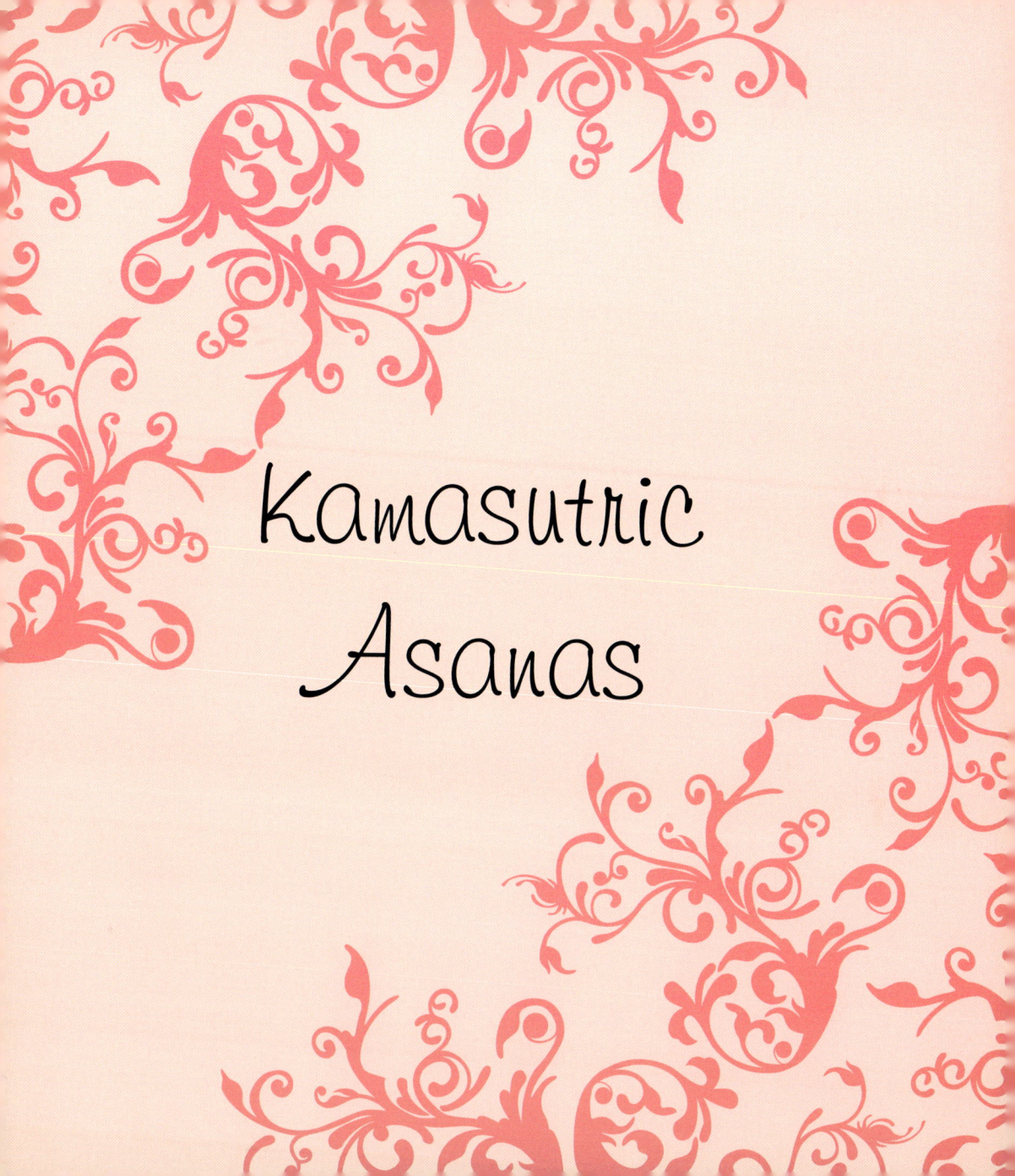

Kamasutric Asanas

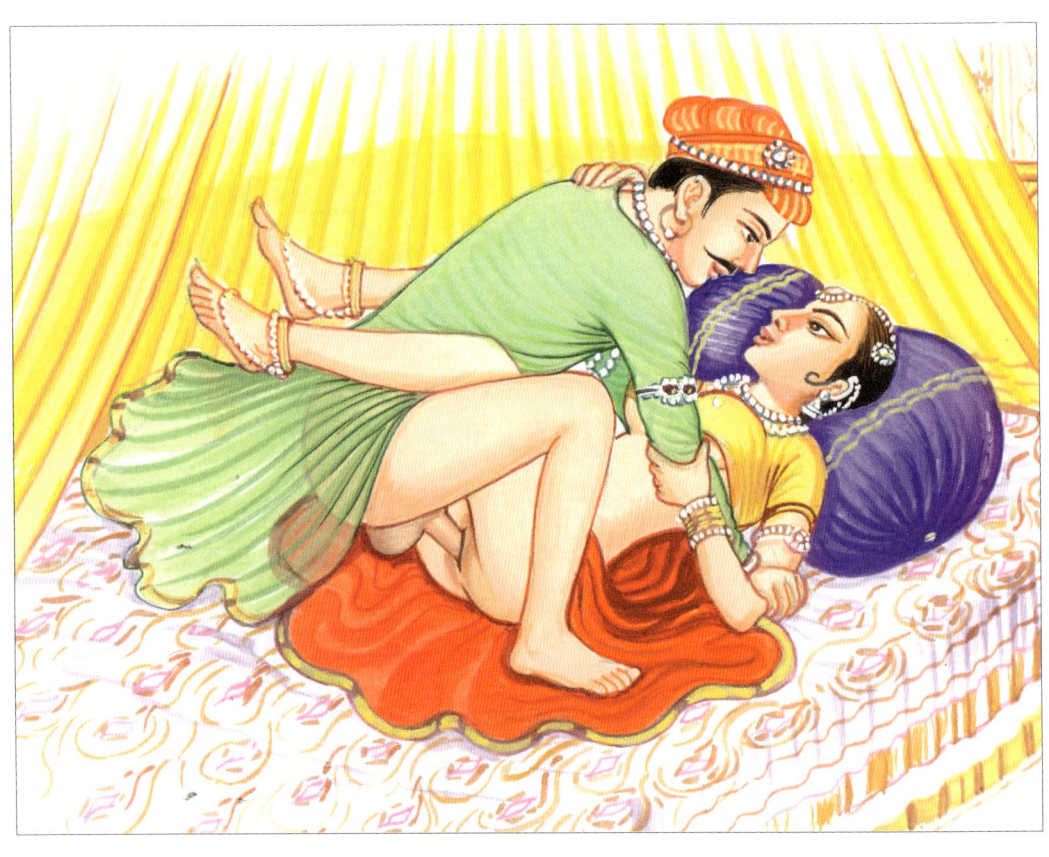

Plate 1 Ab. *Nagara-Uttana-Bandh*

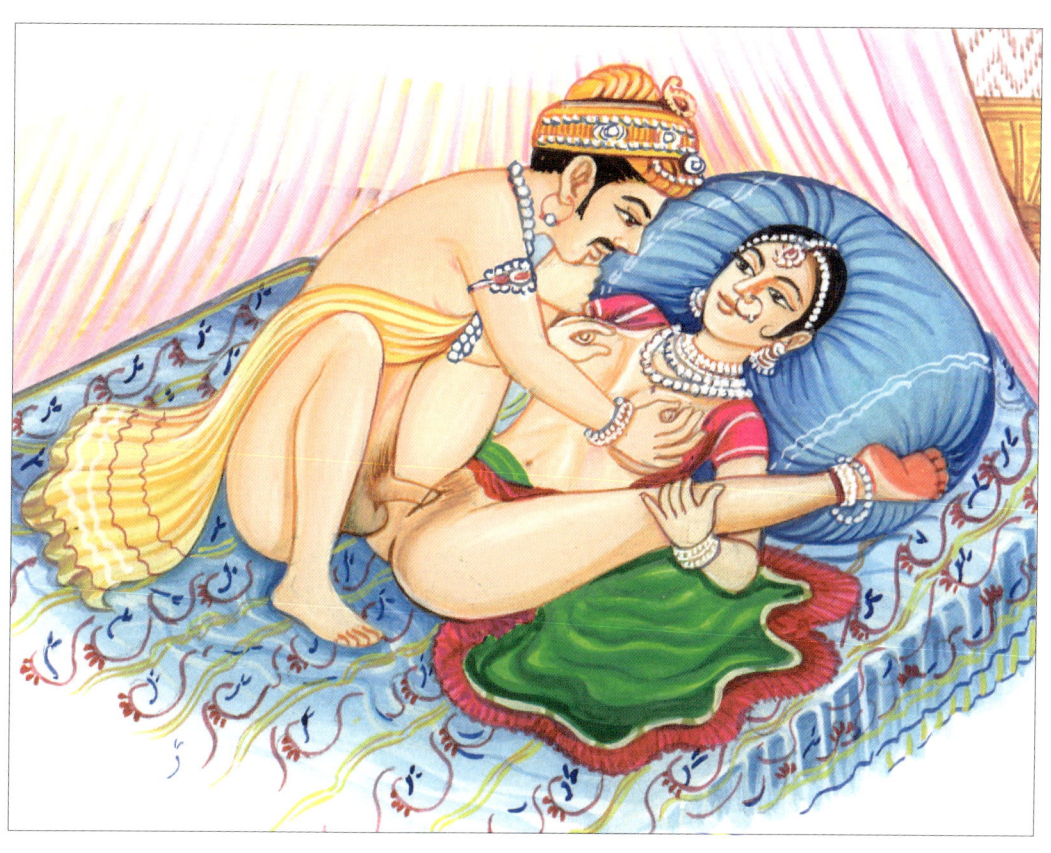

Plate 2 Ad. *Vyompada-Uttana-Bandh*

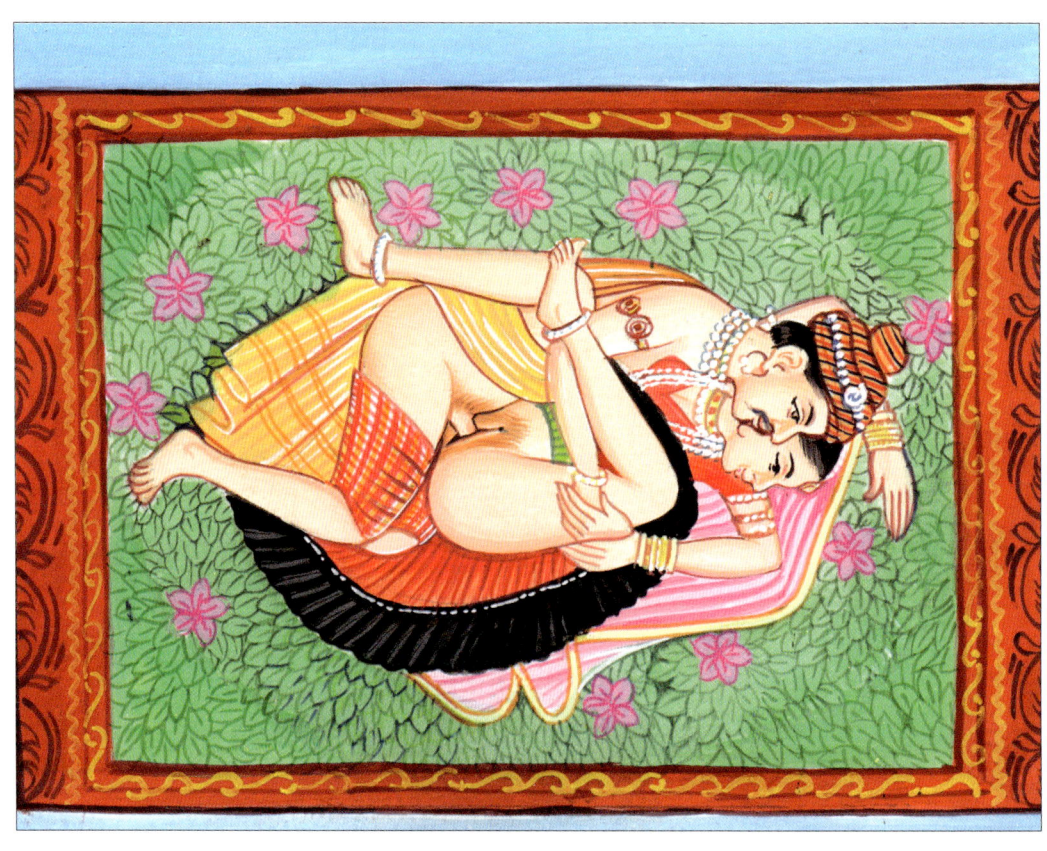

Plate 3 Bb. *Karkata-Tiryak-Bandh*

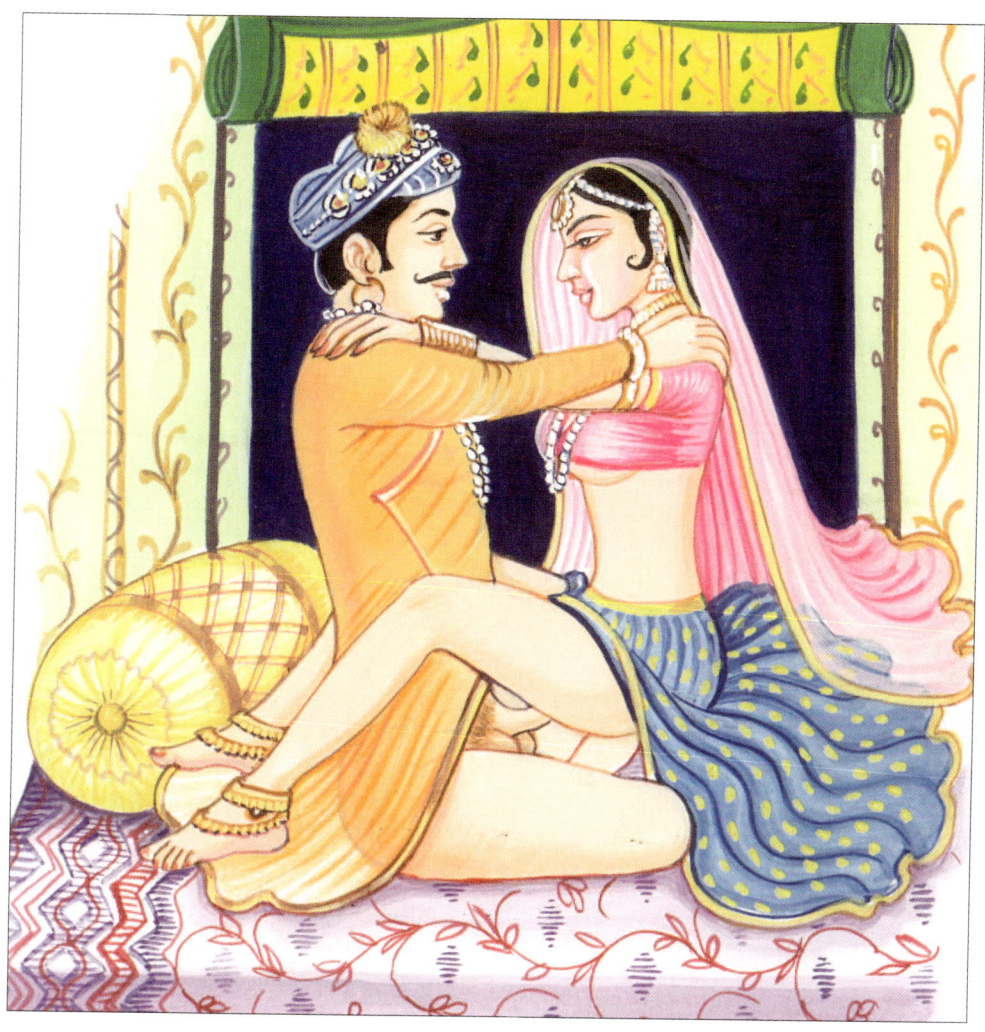

Plate 4 Ca. *Padmasana*

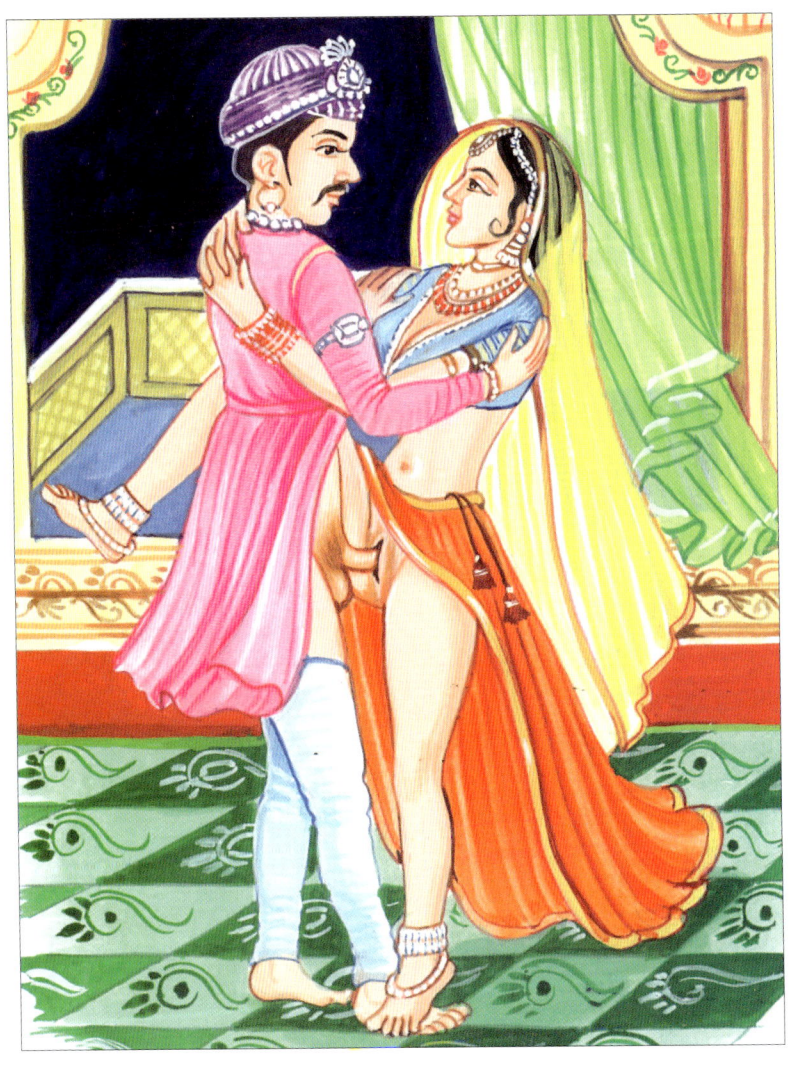

Plate 5 Db. *Hari-Vikrama-Utthita-Bandh*

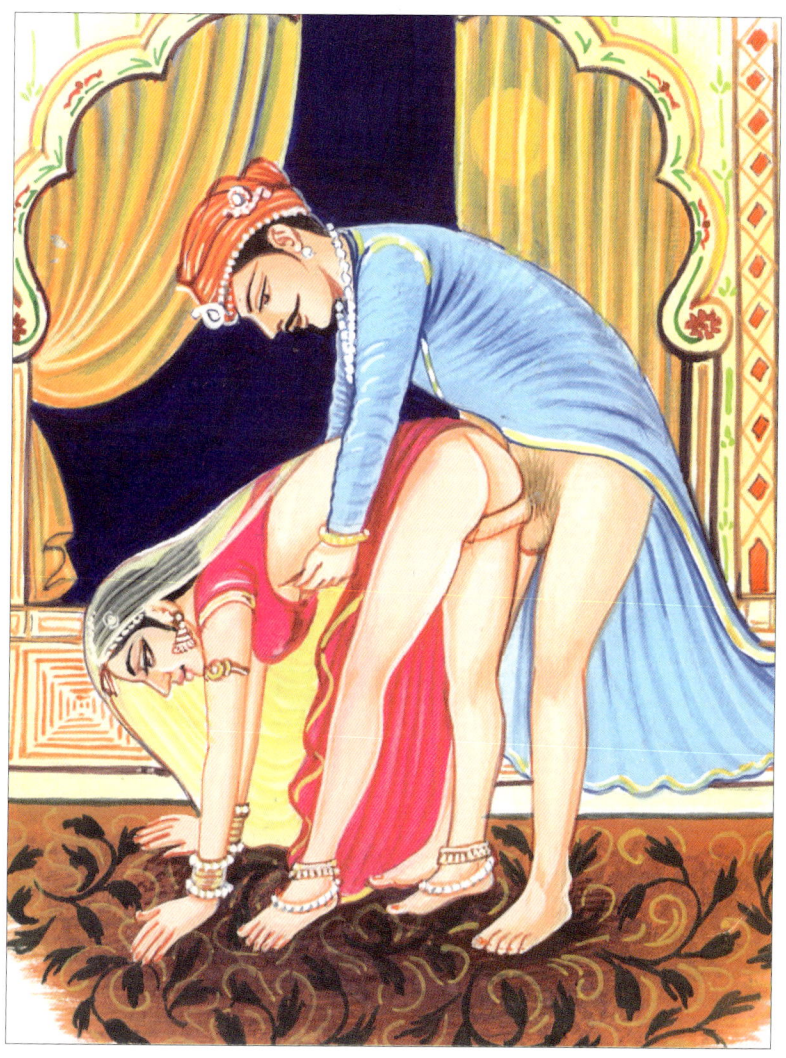

Plate 6 Ea. *Denuka-Vyanta-Bandh*

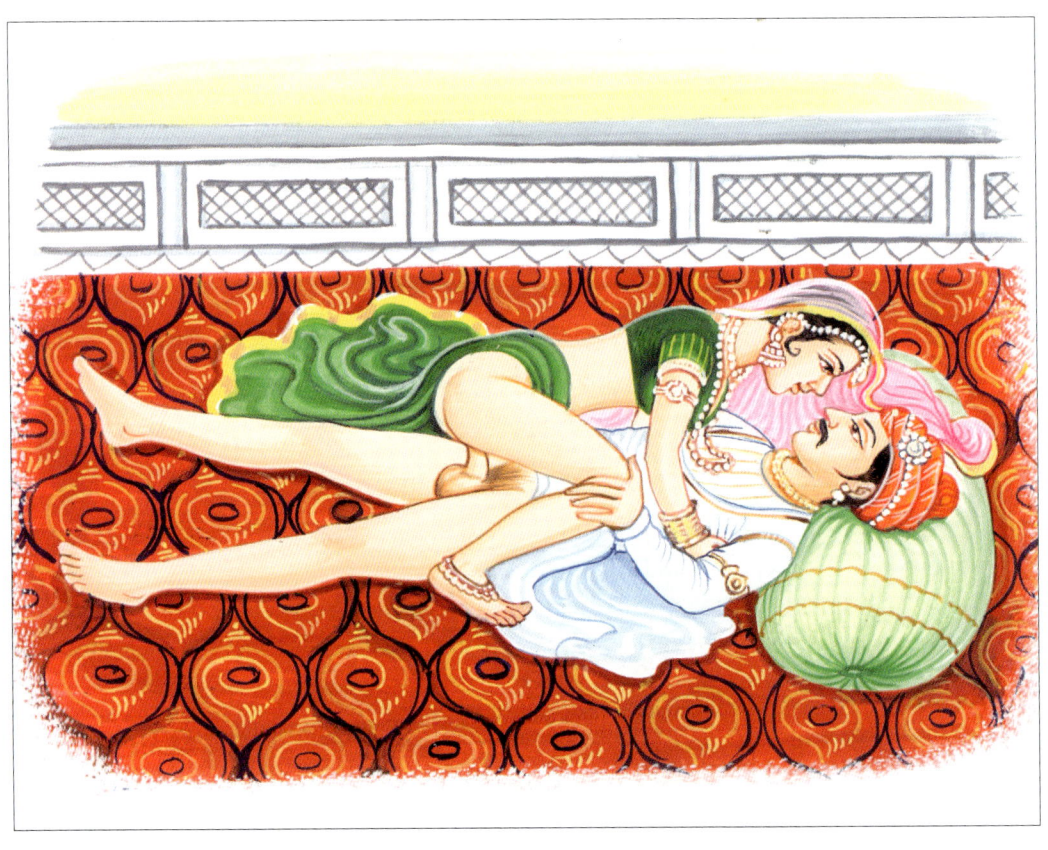

Plate 7 Fa. *Viparita-Bandh*

DIETARY ADVICE

'You are what you eat'
- Albert Signorella

The usual food and drink consumed by an organism is known as 'diet'. However, geographical and dietary diversities make it difficult to discern and standardise a particular diet. But there are a couple of cardinal guidelines that one should always keep in mind and adopt.

- In this unipolar world with Western standardisation more than being prevalent today, a well-balanced diet should contain a sufficient supply of protein, carbohydrates, fats, salts and minerals. The quantity of food absorbed should correspond to the need of the body.

- However, the Eastern concept as regards food and diet – particularly Ayurveda – is different from that of the West and is based on the understanding of the properties of the foods and their effects on the body, rather than their actual constituents.

- One of the ideal 'dietary' systems followed by the Japanese for thousands of years is '**Macrobiotic diet**'. Among its principles are:

    - Eat food that is locally grown or in a similar climate.
    - Include fresh food in daily diet.
    - Select foods in their most natural and whole form and cook lightly.
    - An ideal diet should comprise principle and supplementary foods.
    - At least half (of principle) of one's daily food should consist of wholegrains such as rice, barley, millet, rye and wheat, together with pulses such as lentils and kidney beans.

- Of the supplementary foods, over half should consist of vegetables grown on land and final part could comprise fruits, seafood and meat.
- Steaming and grilling are more preferred cooking methods as opposed to frying.

- Chewing of food more than 18-20 times is most important among all guidelines. Proper chewing and break down of food materials can prevent the onset of a lot of deadly diseases such as diabetes, ulcerations, etc.

'After all don't dig your grave with your knife and fork'
English proverb

- Water consumption needs should also be properly cared for; three-fourth of our earth and more than 70 per cent of our body is water. Hence, always keep the following points in mind:
    - Drink atleast 2 pints or 1-1.5 litres of water everyday, more so when the weather is hot.
    - Slowly sip the water, never gulp.
    - Keep each sip of water in the mouth for a moment, savour, masticate and mix well with saliva.
    - Drink water at room temperature, neither too hot nor too cold.
    - Drink a small quantity at a time but several times a day.
    - A glass of water at bedtime and on getting up in the morning will completely wash the body internally [Ayurveda].
    - Drink water for maintaining proper blood levels, a glowing skin, improved digestion and to get rid of constipation.

To Good Health - Sex...Vigour...Vitality

Following are some simple but effective dietary supplements, most of the time stocked in our kitchen shelves, for vigour, energy and sexuality.

- An excellent aphrodisiac tonic is a combination of onion and honey. Take an onion, peel off the white layer, crush and fry in butter. Eat the mixture on an empty stomach with a spoonful of honey.
- Take forty small red onions, poke these with fork and dip in honey & keep for 40 days. Thereafter take one per day for 40 days.
- Pumpkin/melon seeds, flax, sunflower seeds, cashew and pine nuts also help build sex hormones and are very good for sexual wellbeing.
- Regular consumption of oranges and lemons – antioxidants with vitamin C – protects sex organs, enhances arousal, sensitivity and orgasms.
- Ripe bananas are good for testosterone – male sex hormone – production and libido. These are also rich in potassium and vitamin B.
- Regular use of dates (fruit) soaked in honey strengthens the ovulation process and acts as libido booster. This is an excellent source of iron, too.
- Use of milk boiled with ginger powder after *sambhog* (congress) regenerates the lost power.
- After *sambhog* (congress) use of small quantity of *gur* (jaggery) also makes up quickly for the loss of power and rejuvenates.
- Seeds of watermelon and *mishri* (raw sugar crystals), 5 gms. each taken for 2-3 months makes semen/sperm strong.
- A mixture of onion (white) juice, ginger juice, honey and pure ghee taken in the proportion of 8 gms, 6 gms, 4 gms, and 3 gms respectively, can even cure impotency in two months' time.
- A regular consumption of dark chocolates and caffeine in moderation enhances the sex drive.
- Regular consumption of fish fried in pure ghee is very good to boost libido / orgasm.

pinkyoga

- Diets rich in almonds, olive oil and hazelnuts make men more virile and increases women's sex drive.
- Among seafood, oysters and cavier rich in zinc are good potions and help in production of testosterone.
- Wines, particularly red wines, are supposed to be good aphrodisiacs as they help raise testosterone levels and increase libido.
- Lavish use of ginger and garlic improves the circulatory system and the antioxidants in it protect the body and stir the sexual desire.
- Hot wine flavoured with cardamom is quite an instantaneous enhancer.

Application

- Massage with Jasmine oil on male genitals for 30 minutes everyday for a period of 15 days. It makes the member strong and straight. [**Note:** *Do not apply on front part*]
- For women, pure almond oil massage on breasts turns them shapely and tight.

Acupressure

Acupressure is the art of treating diseases by applying pressure on specific points on the hand/feet (soles) with the help of one's thumb or blunt objects.

Acupressure provides help for
- Prevention of diseases.
- Early diagnosis of diseases.
- Cure of diseases.

Acupressure works on the principles of bioelectricity (current regulations). The flow of electricity (*chetana*) emanates from the 'principle energy'; installed in the body at the time of conception. The flow of current – divided in five zones – passes through the body via the lines called 'meridians'. Starting from the tip of each finger of the right/left hand, the current passes all over the body and ends at the right/left foot, respectively (*see Fig. 3*). As long as the current flows properly throughout the body parts, the body remains fit and healthy. Any interruption in the current flow to any of the points results in the malfunctioning of that part accompanied by pain in some cases. If not attended to in time, it may also invite illness.

Acupressure is the science of nature that teaches us to cure diseases through the inbuilt mechanism of the body by pressure application at corresponding points at palms/soles, thus sending current to all the desired parts of the body.

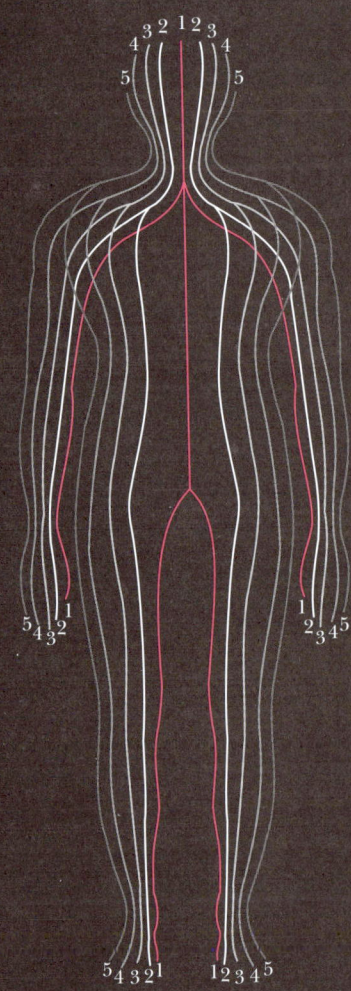

Fig.3 Flow of (Chetana) *electric current-lines*

Acupuncture

Acupuncture is the treatment of pain or disease by inserting the tips of needles at specific points on the skin (about 900 points all over the body on the meridians). Acupressure is also related to acupuncture.

Puncturing is done on these acupressure points to cure illness or pain to create an anaesthetic effect. However, this requires expertise and a good knowledge of the practice. In contrast, acupressure treatment is simple and easy, and anybody can practice the same with a working knowledge of the pressure points.

The Human Body and its Subdivisions

Our body is four dimensional – the right side, the left side, the front and the back. For body parts in the front / back like the spine, nerves, back, lower lumbago, sciatic nerves and hips, pressure is to be applied on the back of the palms / soles (*as shown in Fig. nos. 4 to 7*).

For treatment of organs / parts on the right side of the body the pressure should be administered on the corresponding points of the palm of the right hand or the sole of the right foot and vice-versa on the left side (*as shown in Fig. nos. 8 to 11*).

pinkyoga

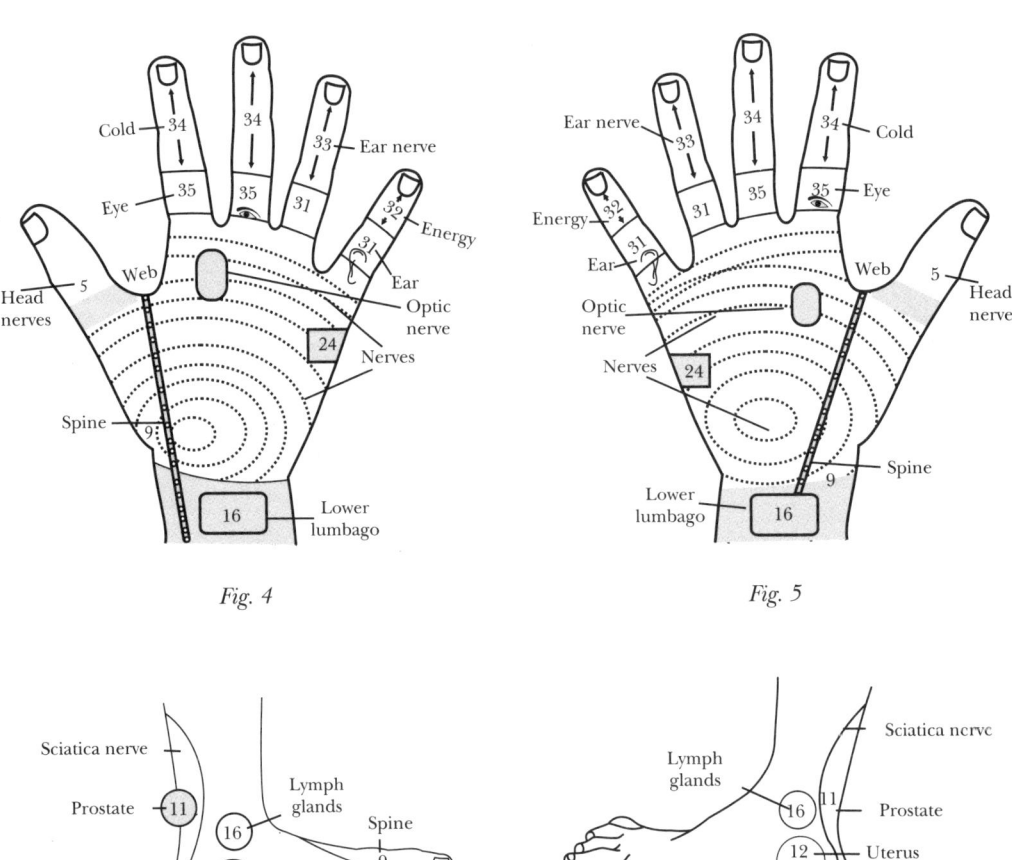

Fig. 4

Fig. 5

Fig. 6

Fig. 7

Pressure Points

1. Brain
2. Mental Nerves
3. Pictuitary Gland
4. Pineal
5. Head Nerves
6. Throat
7. Neck
8. Thyroid and Parathyroid
9. Spine
10. Piles
11. Prostate
12. Uterus
13. Penis/Vagina
14. Ovaries
15. Testes
16. Lymph glands (front) and Lower lumber (back)
17. Hip and Knee
18. Bladder
19. Intestines
20. Colon
21. Appendix
22. Gall Bladder
23. Liver
24. Shoulder
25. Pancreas
26. Kidney
27. Stomach
28. Adrenal
29. Solar Plexus
30. Lungs
31. Ear
32. Energy
33. Nerves and Ear
34. Cold and Nerves
35. Eyes
36. Heart
37. Spleem
38. Thymus

pinkyoga

RIGHT

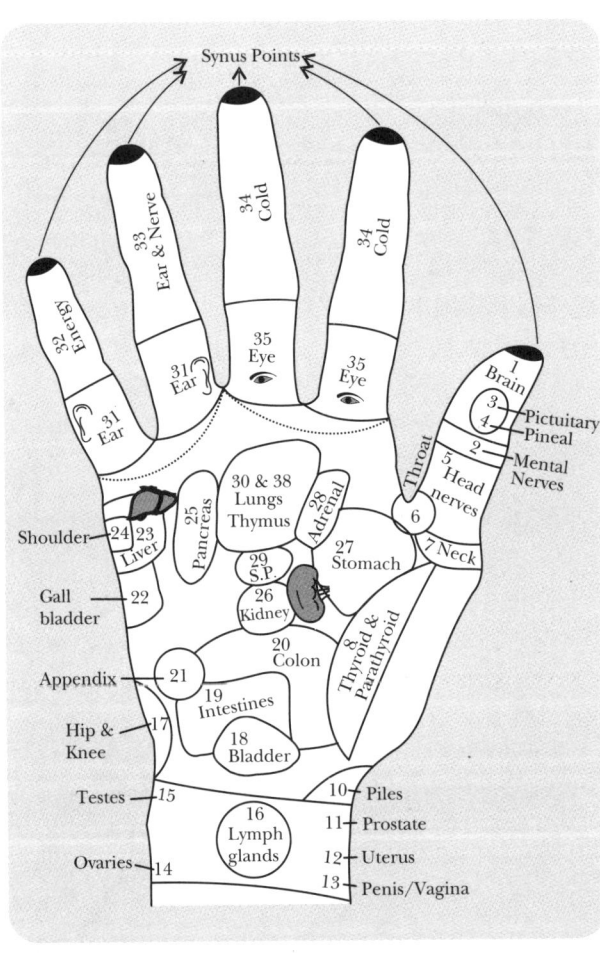

Fig. 8

To Good Health - Sex...Vigour...Vitality

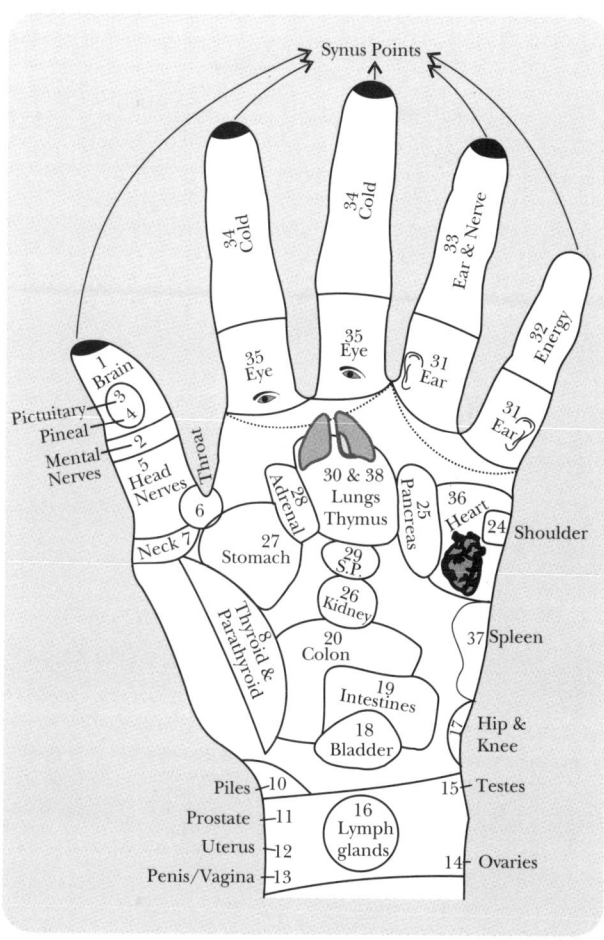

Fig. 9

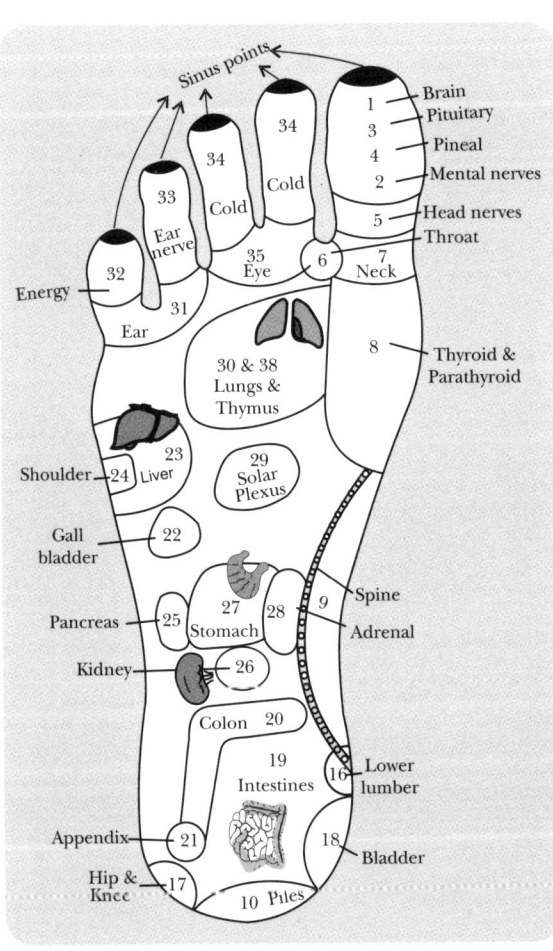

Fig. 10

To Good Health - Sex...Vigour...Vitality

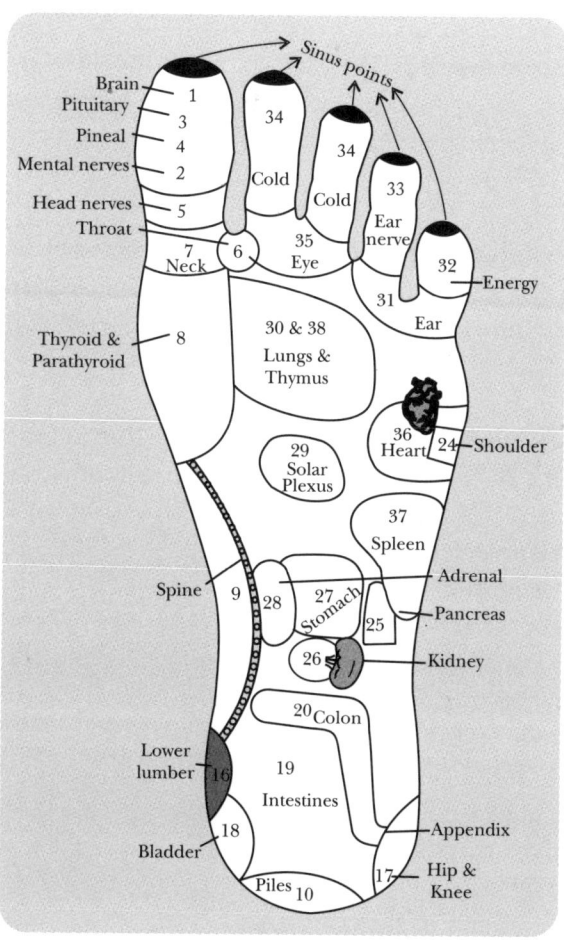

Fig. 11

Treatment

How much pressure to be applied – The pressure applied should be just enough for you to be able to feel it. However, on all the points of the endocrine glands, deeper pressure is to be applied by keeping the thumb vertical, whereas on all other points it (thumb) is to be kept horizontal.

What should be the duration of pressure – For the treatment of any disease / organ, pressure should be applied, in fact intermittent pressure like pumping for 2-3 minutes at a time, and should be repeated three times a day. The treatment should be continued till the pain on that point subsides.

What time of the day can this method be practised – The acupressure treatment can be taken any time during the 24 hours; but it is advisable to avoid it within one hour of the meals.

What is the anaesthetic effect – If continued pressure is applied for more than three minutes, it creates an anaesthetic effect on the organ connected with it. For the points on fingers, cloth pins or rubber bands can be used (*as shown in Fig. 12*). In case the tips of the fingers or toes become blue, remove the pressure. Such continued pressure on the corresponding points is very useful during severe headache, stomach ache, etc. For toothache, continuous pressure is to be applied on the tips of the fingers relating to that particular tooth (*see Fig. 13*).

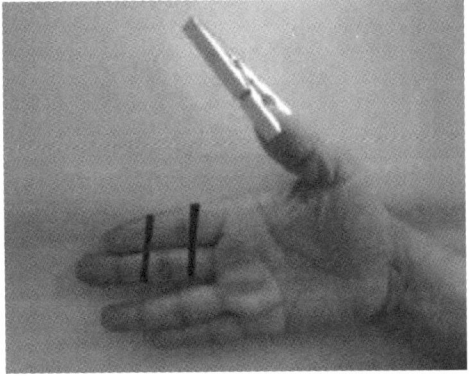

Fig. 12

To Good Health - Sex...Vigour...Vitality

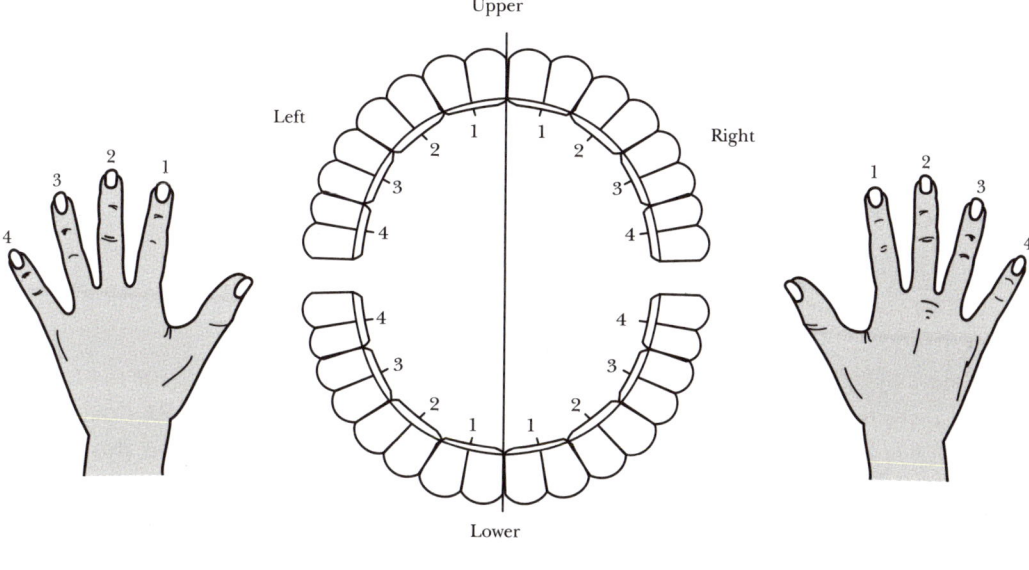

Fig. 13

Precaution

Please do not continue pressing the points for longer durations during the day in the hope of an early cure, as this may damage the points (switches). Unnecessary prolonging the pressure may cause damage to the kidneys due to extra release of toxins in the body.

> **NOTE:** *At the end of every session kidney points should also be treated as a regular habit.*

Side effects

- The important feature of this treatment is that there are no side effects. The treatment is harmless and can be safely given even to a one-day-old child.

A Holistic Treatment

As a layman, our objective is to diagnose and get rid of the disease through accupressure. In this regard, it is advisable to adopt a routine of daily massage of palms / soles atleast 2-3 minutes a day, preferably by applying few drops of oil. If any point pains / hurts then press the point – in a pumping manner – for 2 minutes and repeat this treatment three times in 24 hours. **This treatment is to be continued only till you feel pain on that point. When the pain is removed, the disease is also removed with it and you are cured. THIS TREATMENT IS TO BE STOPPED THEN AND CONTINUE WITH THE ROUTINE ONE.**

Thus:
- Daily 10 minutes of pressing palms / soles helps **prevention** of the disease setting in.
- Once hurting point(s) are located, the **diagnosis** is facilitated.
- Special /extra treatment thereafter helps to **cure** the problem.

[**Note:** *The science of acupressure is believed to do miracles as it is based on bioelectricity. The relief at times could be faster than even the effect of an injection*].

5

Therapeutic Applications and Common Problems

'Before you have practised, the theory is useless. After you have practised, the theory is obvious.'
- **David Williams**

The following table helps in identifying the ailment and understanding the types of *asanas/pranayama*, acupressure treatment associated with it for complete cure of the disease. A list of do's and dont's has also been provided for reference.

The sequence to follow these regimes should be *asanas* followed by *pranayamas* and then acupressure. If the time available is less, then the acupressure regime could be spread over the day's routine.

A very beneficial massage, quite useful for quick relief is the **APM (acu-press-massage)**. Use a few drops of oil and massage both the palms and back of the palms with little pressure to locate pain, if any; thus achieving automatic and advance diagnosis of impending problem(s) and at the same time giving treatment, too.

Therapeutic

S. NO.	DISORDER/DISEASES	ASANAS/PRANAYAM	ACUPRESSURE	CAUTION/REMARKS
1.	Arthritis/ Rheumatic Diseases/ Gout	A:Shavasana->S. Namaskar ->Bhujanga->Shalabha->Viprita-karni->Matsya->Shavasana. P: Anulom Vilom (AV) ->Kapalbhati->Naad->AV.	APM+tips of fingers and toes + sciatica points	High BP/ cervical spondylitis patients to avoid Vipritakarni.
2.	Asthma (lungs)/ Respiratory	A: Surya Namaskar->Shavasana->Ushtra->Vajra->Gomukh-> Shashanka->Matsya->Shavasana P: AV->Ujjayi->Kapalbhati->Naad->AV	1 to 7+ 21+ 30+ 34	No holding of breath during asanas/ pranayama
3.	Cervical Spondylitis/ Backache	A: Tada+Ushtra+Vajra+ Supta Vajra- >Shashanka- >Bhujanga-> Shalabha->Kandhara ->Matsya->Shavasana. P: AV->Kapalbhati->Naad->AV.	APM+1 to 7+ +16	
4.	Constipation	A: Surya Namaskar->Shavasana ->Tada->Vajra->SuptaVajra-> Shashanka->Bhujanga->Shalabha-> Matsya->Shavasana. P: AV->Kapalbhati->Naad->AV.	APM	High BP/cervical spondylitis patients avoid Surya Namaskar
5.	Diabetes	A: Surya Namaskar -+Shavasana [-and/or-]->Vajra-> Supta Vajra-> Shashanka->Vakra-> Vipritakarni ->Matsya->Shavasana. P: AV->Kapalbhati->Naad->AV	APM+25+26.	Observe cautions cited above as required.

Therapeutic Applications and Common Problems

S. NO.	DISORDER/DISEASES	ASANAS/PRANAYAM	ACUPRESSURE	CAUTION/REMARKS
6.	ENT- Ear, Nose and Throat	A: Ushtrasana->Vajra->Vakra->Bhujanga->Shalabha->Vipritakarni->Matsya->Shavasana. P: AV->Ujjayi->Naad->AV.	APM+ 6+7+8+31 to 35.	
7.	Gastric (indigestion)	A: Surya Namaskar+Shavasana [-and/or-HVajra->SuptaVajra->Shashanka->Bhujanga->Shalabha-> -►Shavasana. P: AV->Kapalbhati->AV.	APM+19+22+23 +27.	
8.	Headache	A: Vajra->Vakra->Bhujanga->Shalabha->Vipritakarni->->Matsya->Shavasana. P: AV->Naad->Ujjayi->Kapalbhati->AV.	APM+ (a) 1 to 7+34 (b) 22+23+25+26.	(A) If due to cold. (B) If due to heat.
9.	Heart	Initially for the first three weeks, only morning and evening walks followed by Tadasana and Shavasana. In addition do AV in Gyan Mudra and APM. Thereafter: A: Vajra->Gomukha->Bhujanga-> Shalabha->Matsya->Shavasana. P: AV->Ujjayi->Naad->AV.	APM + 36 twice a day.	Refer to caution at S.NO. 2
10.	Hernia	A: Shavasana+Tadasana+Vajra->SuptaVajra->Shashanka->Matsya->Shavasana. P: AV->Naad->AV.	APM+11 to 15.	(A) If in advance stages; surgical intervention should be solicited. (B) Eat light and easily digestible food.

83

S. NO.	DISORDER/DISEASES	ASANAS/PRANAYAM	ACUPRESSURE	CAUTION/REMARKS
11.	BP (High)	A: Vajra+SuptaVajra+ Shashanka->Bhujanga -> Shalabha-> Shavasana (prolonged) P: AV->Ujjayi->Naad-> Kapalbhati->AV.	APM+3+4+8 +14+15+25+28	Refer to caution at S.NO. 2 .
12.	BP (low)	A: Surya Namaskar+ all asanas of high BP (above). P: As for high BP (above).	APM+4+22+23 +25+28.	Same as for high B P.
13.	Insomnia/ Nervousness	A: Surya Namaskar+ Shavasana+Ushtra+Vajra+ SuptaVajra->Shashanka-> Viparitakarani Matsya - ▶ Shavasana. P: AV+Kapalbhati->Naad->AV. ->30 minutes of Yoga Nidra	APM + Clasp your hands tightly interlocking the fingers. Then with fingers of the left hand press on the back of the right hand and vice versa for 1-2 minutes. Practice 3-4 times a day.	Consult a biochemist doctor for course of Kali Phos. (Bio chemic medicine)
14.	Liver	A: Ushtra+Vajra ->SuptaVajra->Shashanka-> Vakra->Matsya->Shavasana. P: AV->Kapalbhati->Naad->AV.	APM+22+23+25 +26.	
15.	Menstrual	A: Vajra+Gomukha+SuptaVajra ->Shashanka->Bhujanga-> Shalabha->Matsya->Shavasana. P: AV->Kapalbhati->Naad->AV.	APM+11 to 15 +26	

Therapeutic Applications and Common Problems

S. NO.	DISORDER/DISEASES	ASANAS/PRANAYAM	ACUPRESSURE	CAUTION/REMARKS
16.	Obesity	A: Surya Namaskar+Shavasana ->Vajra-> SuptaVajra-> Shashanka->Gomukha-> Bhujanga->Shalabha -> Viparitakarani->Matsya -▶Shavasana. P: AV->Kapalbhati->Naad->AV	APM+3+4+8+11 to 15+22+23+ 25+28+26.	Chew food properly; consume liquids atleast 18-20 times a day; never swallow.
17.	Piles	A: Surya Namaskar (slow and rhythmically) + Asanas of S.No. 4 (Constipation) P: same as for constipation	APM+10	Get rid of constipation by medicine and solar plexus correction, if required.
18.	Pyelitis (Kidney)	A:Vajra->SuptaVajra-> Shashanka->Gomukh->Vakra-> Bhujanga->Shalabha->'-> Matsya->Shavasana. P: AV->Kapalbhati->Naad->AV.	APM+26	Chew food properly; consume liquids atleast 18-20 times a day; never swallow.
19.	Sperm/ Virility	A: Vajra->SuptaVajra-> Shashanka+GomukhaVakra^ Bhujanga->Shalabha-> Viparitakarani->Matsya-> Shavasana. P: AV->Kapalbhati->AV.	APM+11 to 15	
20.	Urinary/ Stones	A: SuryaNamaskar +Shavasana [-and/or-] -> Vakra ->Bhujanga-> Shalabha ->Viparitakarani-> Matsya -> Shavasana. P: AV->Kapalbhati->Naad->AV.	APM+8+11 to 15+26	

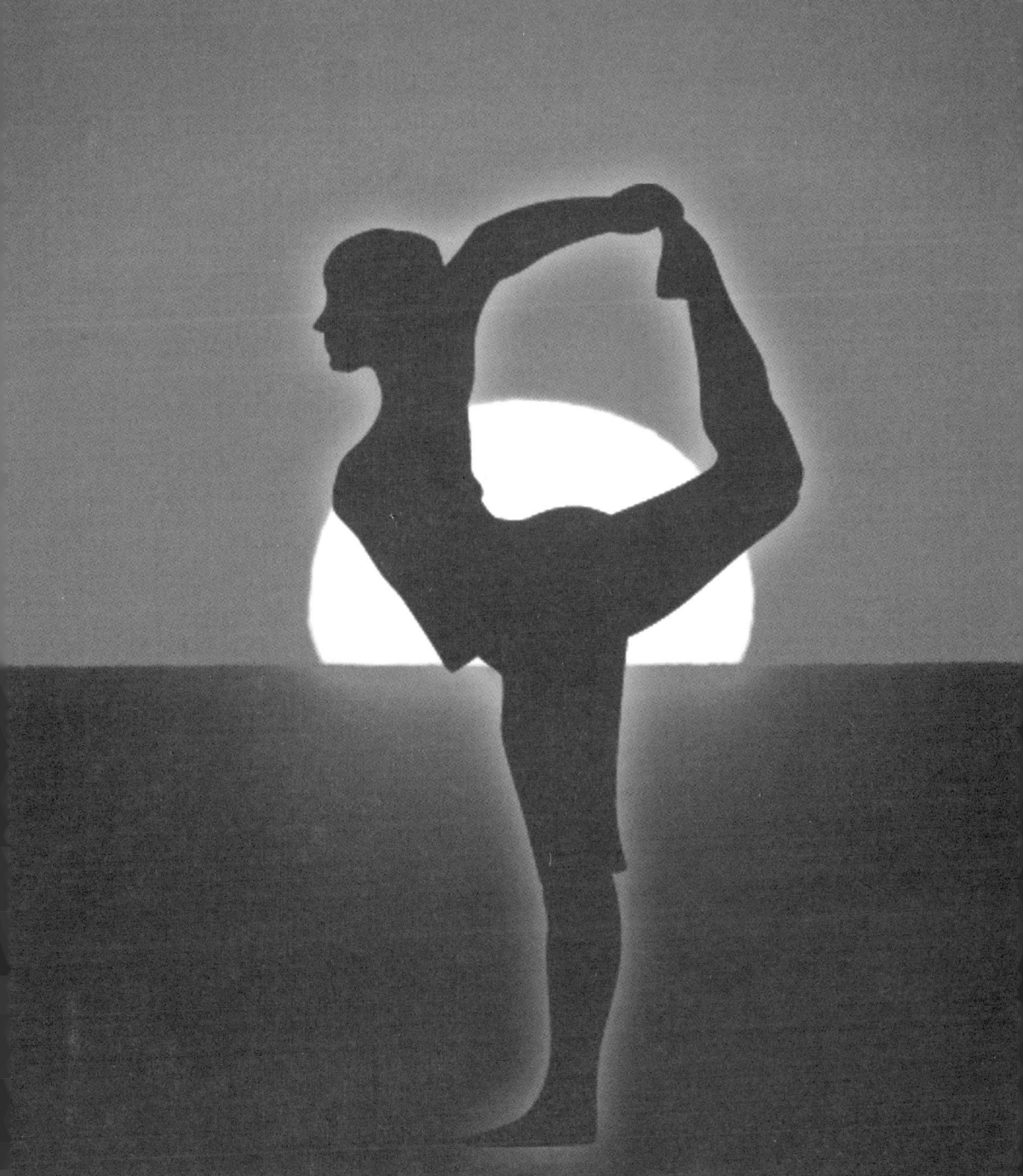

6

Ideal Packages

This chapter deals with 'ideal packages' for different age groups, to derive adequate benefits to maintain good health. But if therapeutic essentialities are there; one must add more *asanas / pranayama*, etc., to derive optimum benefits.

Also the duration of these packages are for normal health maintenance/well-being. The duration would have to be increased if some problems continue to exist. These would, however, require an additional yogic therapy.

Basically, three packages are discussed hereafter:
- I - Package (age group 13-30 yrs)
- II - Package (age group 30-45 yrs)
- III - Package (age group 45 and above)

[**Note:** *Yoga below 13 yrs of age is not recommended*].

I - Package (age group 13-30 yrs)
- ***Asanas:*** (20 mins.)
    - Shavasana (2 mins.) + Surya Namaskar (3-5 sets) + Vajra + Gomukha + Suptavajra + Shashanka + Viparitakarani + Matsya + Tada + Shavasana
- ***Pranayamas:*** (10 mins.)
    - Anulom Vilom (**AV**) + Ujjayi + Naad + AV
- ***Acupressure:*** (5 mins.)
    - Acupressure Massage (**APM**)

II - Package (age group 30-45 yrs)
- *Asanas:* (20 mins.)
  - Shavasana+ Surya Namaskar (2-3 sets) Vajra + Gomukha + Vakra +Bhujanga Shalabha + Viparitkarani + Matsya + Tadasana + Shavasana
- *Pranayamas:* (15 mts.)
  - AV + Ujjayi + Kapalbhati + Naad + AV
- *Acupressure:* APM

III - Package (age group 45 yrs and above)
- *Asanas:* (25 mins.)
  - Shavasana + Surya Namaskar (1-2 set) Ushtrasana + Vajra + S.Vajra Kandhara Matsya Tada Shavasana
- *Pranayamas:* (15 mins.)
  - AV + Ujjayi + Kapalbhati + Naad + AV
- *Acupressure:* APM

Important Notes:
- The practitioner is advised to fine tune the packages from earlier chapters on *asanas / pranayamas*, etc. and also increase / decrease the duration to suit individual body and time availability.
- If suffering from high B.P. or spine problems, please do not practice *Surya Namaskar*, instead do *Ushtrasan*.
- Those suffering from hernia are not to practice *Bhujanga / Shalabhasana*.
- The Acupressure durations may be spread over the day if there are time constraints during regular yogic sessions.

Acknowledgements

1. Swami Vivekananda – Analysis and Scriptures on Patanjali '*Yog Sutras*' & '*Raj Yoga*'.
2. Padmashri Bharat Bhushan, Yogacharya, Saharanpur.
3. Swami Kuvalayananda (Founder Director of Scientific Institute for Yoga Research, Lonavla, Pune, India).
4. Devendra Vora, Mumbai – Publications of Acupressure and other Natural therapies.
5. Swami Sivananda – Divine Life Society, Rishikesh, India.
6. Bhartiya Yog Sansthan.
7. Swami Ramdev (*Divya Yog Sansthan*, Haridwar India).
8. Dr Phulgendra Sinha (Director Institutes of Yoga, Patna, India & Washington, USA).
9. *Kamasutra* (of Vatsayayan) - Sir Richard Burton.
10. *And my technical advisors:* **KG Agarwal; Dr DJ Sen Gupta, MBBS, MDerma; Vijay Agarwal and Miloosha Sharma.**

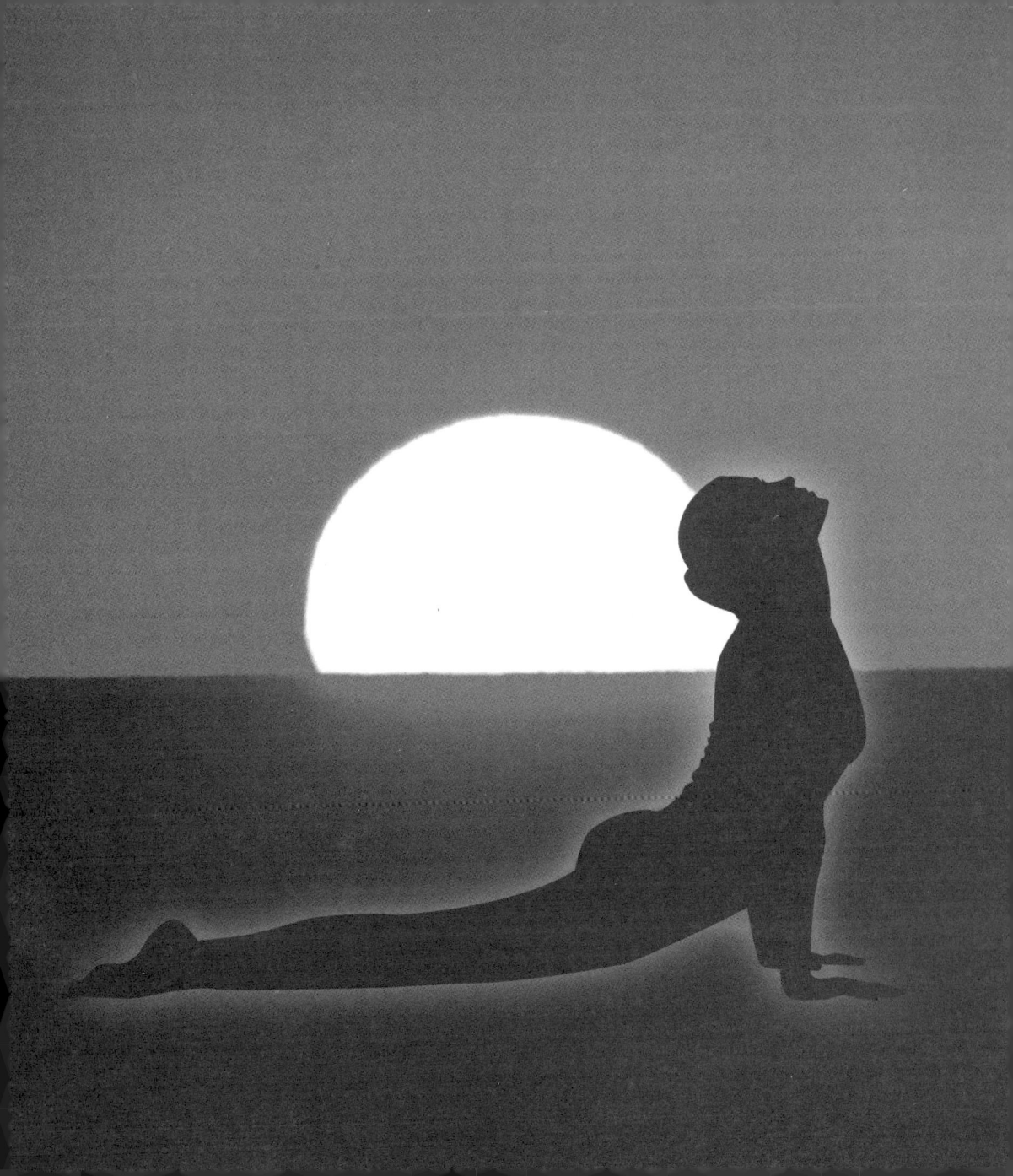

Index

Note: The letters 'f' following locators denote figures.

A

Acupressure, 69–80
  acupuncture, 71
  anaesthetic effect, 78
  holistic treatment, 80
  human body and its subdivisions, 71
  'meridians', 69
  precaution, 79
  pressure points, 73
  pressure, duration, 78
  principles of bioelectricity, 69
  side effects, 80
  treatment, 78
AIDS (Acquired Immuno Deficiency Syndrome), 11–12
APM (acu-press-massage), 81
Ashtang Yoga, 13–14
Ayurveda, 65

B

Bandhs (Air Locks), 45–47
  Jalandhara Bandh, 45
  Maha Bandh, 47
  Moola Bandh, 47
  Uddiyana Bandh, 46
Bhoga (physical pleasure), 56
Bhujangasana (Cobra pose), 31
Brihadaranyaka Upanishad, 56

C

Cerebro spinal fluid, 12
Chetana (electric current-lines), flow chart, 70*f*

D

Dietary advice, 64–68
  application, 68
  dietary supplements, 67–68
  eastern concept, 65
  macrobiotic diet, 65–66
  principles, 65
  proper chewing of food, 66
  western standardisation, 65

E

Electromagnetic field around the body, 7
'Emotional tree', 6*f*, 10, 13
'Emotion-booster-cum-tranquiliser', 10
Emotions, 6
'Emotions' and 'hormonal secretions', 7

G

Gomukhasana (Cow's Face pose), 27
Guidelines for practitioners before starting yoga, 14–16

H

Healthy and relaxed mind, 9
Hectic lifestyle, 9
Human body, 3

I

Ida Nadi, 36
Ideal Packages, 87–88
  Package I (age group 13–30 yrs), 88
  Package II (age group 30–45 yrs), 88
  Package III, (age group 45 yrs and above), 88

K

Kamasutra, 2, 55
Kamasutric Art of Love, 55–64
  external enjoyments, 58
  Grahastha ashrama, 57
  guidelines, 64
  internal enjoyments, 59–64
  Kamasanas, 59
  male and female, classification of, 57–58

Purushayita Bandh, 63
theories of *kama*, 57
Tiryaka, 61
Upavishta (Sitting Posture), 62
Uttana Bandha, 60–61
Utthita, 62
Vyanta-Bandh (Cow Posture), 63
Kandharasana (Cave posture), 32
Konark and Khajuraho, 56
Kundalini, 7, 12

'Material Survival', 6
Matsyasana (Fish pose), 35
Meditation, 48–51
    dharana: dhyan: samadhi, 49
    indriya-centric meditation, 49
    movement meditation, 51
    vibration meditation, 50
Moksha, 56
Mooladhar chakra, 7, 10, 37

Nectar, 13

Nirvana (salvation), 56
'No-time-for-anything' attitude, 9

OM, auspicious sounds, *see* also Meditation

Padmasana (Lotus pose), 19
Pain treatment by inserting the needles, *see* Acupuncture
Perversion tendencies, 13
Pingala Nadi, 37
Pranayama – Breath Control, 36–42
    Types of, 37–42
    Alternative Kapalbhati, 41
    Anulom Vilom / Nadi Shodhan, 38–39
    Kapalbhati, 41
    Naad Yoga, 42
    Ujjayi, 40
Prolonged concentration, 49, *see* also Meditation

Psychological lust, 9
Puberty, beginning of, 11

Reproductive biology, 12

Samadhi, 49, *see* also Meditation
Semen, formation process, 11
Sequence during yogic session, 16
Sex hormonal secretions (SHS), 1, 7
Shalabhasana (Locust pose), 33
Shashankasana (Face down Hero's pose), 29
Shavasana (Corpse pose), 18
'Spinning wheels of energy', 35
'Spirituality', 6
Sukhasana (Comfortable pose), 20
Supta Vajrasana (Hero's pose in lying position), 28
Surya Namaskar (Sun Salutation), 22–25
Sushumna Nadi, 37

Swadhisthan chakras, 10

Tadasana (Stretch pose), 21
Therapeutic Applications, 81–85

Vajrasana (Hero's pose), 26
Vakrasana (Spinal Twist pose), 30
Vatsayayan, 2, 55
Viparitakarani (Inverted posture), 34

Warm bath, 16
Water consumption, 66

Yoga (spiritual exercise), 56
Yoga Nidra: Yogic Sleep, 43–44